41 10

LIFT

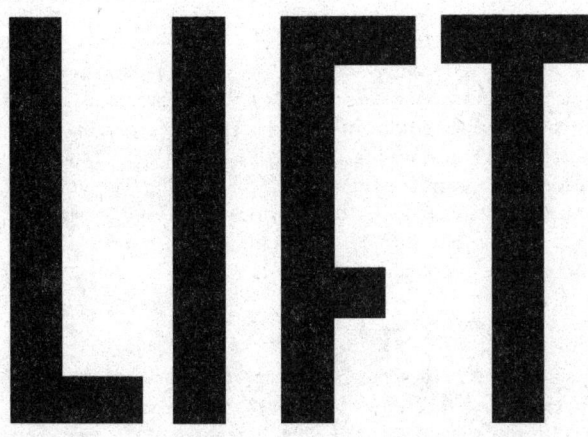

LIFT

How Women Can Reclaim Their Physical Power
and Transform Their Lives

Anne Marie Chaker

AVERY
AN IMPRINT OF PENGUIN RANDOM HOUSE
NEW YORK

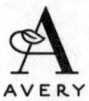

AVERY

an imprint of Penguin Random House LLC
1745 Broadway, New York, NY 10019
penguinrandomhouse.com

Avery with colophon is a trademark of Penguin Random House LLC

Most Avery books are available at a discount when purchased in quantity for sales promotions or corporate use. Special editions, which include personalized covers, excerpts, and corporate imprints, can be created when purchased in large quantities. For more information, please e-mail specialmarkets@penguinrandomhouse.com. Your local bookstore can also assist with discounted bulk purchases using the Penguin Random House corporate Business-to-Business program. For assistance in locating a participating retailer, e-mail B2B@penguinrandomhouse.com.

Illustration on page 196 by Ihor Biliavskyi / Shutterstock

Book design by Ashley Tucker

Library of Congress Cataloging-in-Publication Data

Names: Chaker, Anne Marie, author.
Title: Lift: how women can reclaim their physical power and transform their lives / Anne Marie Chaker.
Description: New York: Avery, an imprint of Penguin Random House, 2025. | Includes index.
Identifiers: LCCN 2024044692 (print) | LCCN 2024044693 (ebook) | ISBN 9780593541111 (hardcover) | ISBN 9780593541135 (epub)
Subjects: LCSH: Weight training for women. | Physical fitness for women. | Women—Mental health. | Body image in women.
Classification: LCC GV546.6.W64 C46 2025 (print) | LCC GV546.6.W64 (ebook) | DDC 613.7/13082—dc23/eng/20250203
LC record available at https://lccn.loc.gov/2024044692
LC ebook record available at https://lccn.loc.gov/2024044693

Printed in the United States of America
1st Printing

The authorized representative in the EU for product safety and compliance is Penguin Random House Ireland, Morrison Chambers, 32 Nassau Street, Dublin D02 YH68, Ireland, https://eu-contact.penguin.ie.

For my mother,
Louise Langlois Chaker,
Who embodies strength

For my daughters,
Juliette and Sylvie,
Who follow in her footsteps

And for Rick,
The love of my life

CONTENTS

Strength should be an attribute of all humanity. It's not a gift that belongs solely to the male of the species.

Jan Todd, first woman to deadlift more than 400 pounds in 1976

People used to say that if women worked out, they would become masculine-looking or wouldn't be able to get pregnant. We just laughed because we knew they were wrong.

Abbye "Pudgy" Stockton, organizer of the first Amateur Athletic Union–sanctioned weightlifting competition for women in 1947

There is no perfect time. No perfect opportunity. No perfect situation. No perfect moment. You either make it happen, or you don't. You don't wait for it to fall in your lap. You take it.

Mattie Rogers, World Weightlifting Championships silver medalist 2017, 2019, 2021, and 2022

INTRODUCTION

In late 2014, I entered a tough phase in my life. My second daughter was born in December, and I was reeling from the effects of postpartum depression, barely sleeping, feeling anxious and unhinged. Two weeks later, my father, who lived a few doors down from my house, died suddenly of a heart attack. The months that followed were a blur. Weekly visits to a marriage counselor with my husband weren't leading to the greater intimacy I had hoped for. What started as nightly half glasses of wine to take the edge off turned into full-bottle binges. Food was an afterthought—it was whatever I consumed between morning coffee and evening wine, the stuff that came off my children's plates. I was treating my body like a waste bin. I went on like this for months, and then months became two years. I hated the reflection in the mirror: I looked bloated and sad. I hit a low point when I took a work call one Friday at four p.m. and could hear myself slurring words.

I realized that it was time for a change one weekend in February 2019. That Saturday, I climbed in my car to drive my eldest daughter, who was nearly eight at the time, to her ice hockey tournament. I'd recently signed up as a volunteer coach on her team, so I packed up the Subaru with my coaching gear, her hockey gear, and a stroller for the toddler. My husband had moved out a few months earlier, and single-parenting was very new, so my mother joined on the passenger's side; the idea was she'd watch the little one while I coached. Here I was, hoping to be a good role model for the girls on my daughter's team, all ages eight and under, who were already receiving plenty of messages, implicitly and explicitly, that they didn't belong. As a Mom Coach, I was getting similarly snubbed by the Dad Coaches on the ice. Armed with my hockey skates and whistle, I was attempting to prove to the boys and their dads that women and girls belonged in this sport, too, that we were strong and deserving. But as I pulled away with my mother at my side and the kids in the back, I had the most powerful feeling, like an itch I desperately needed to scratch: I needed a drink. I could not wait to hit the hotel mini-bar. I knew something needed to give; I just didn't know what.

At some point not long after we arrived at the hotel, checked in, and dropped our bags in the room, I noticed there was a small fitness area. I hadn't entered any kind of gym in a long time. I was barely exercising—attempting a jog here and there after the guilt from a binge of Doritos and sauvignon blanc. At the age of forty-two, I was still reeling from bringing two babies into the world—I didn't have anything that would constitute a workout routine. I'm not sure what possessed me to wander into the hotel gym, but that's where I saw her: a petite blond woman in black shorts and a white racerback shirt lifting barbells and dumbbells and pulling on resistance bands. She looked youthful and her muscles popped when she exercised, reminding me of my rowing teammates in the college weight room more than two decades earlier. I also noticed she logged in her results on her phone. Her face was sweaty and determined, but also nonplussed, as if she had done this a thousand times and knew what she was doing. The combination of her know-how and superhero physique was intriguing to me.

I got up the nerve to introduce myself. She told me her name was Sara, and it turned out her daughter was on the team I coached. I asked what sport or fitness regimen she followed. When she said she did bikini competitions, I tried not to laugh. She explained that this was part of the sport of bodybuilding, how she would get onstage and compete against other women in a bikini, and how her meal planning was entirely measured by "macros"—macronutrients. I was amused but also intrigued by the discipline it must take and the knowledge she must have acquired from her training.

When I was younger, I'd considered myself an athlete, even if, somehow, my body had never quite fit with whichever sport I tried. In high school, I was a figure skater, until I realized that I didn't have that ballerina-svelte frame that the advanced girls all seemed to have. In college, I discovered rowing, which meant I also started lifting weights to get strong enough to compete. Soon enough, I got bumped from my seat on the boat for being too short, but continued to work out at the gym, at least while I was still at school. After I graduated, and there weren't any more team meets or practices to attend, athletics disappeared into the distance. That construct—coach, team, practice schedule—was replaced by the unpredictable mess of life, which included student loans, rent to pay, bosses, and deadlines. If I did exercise, it was always as a kind of punishment for overindulging, to try to make myself thinner. Being connected to my body—let alone pushing it to attain some sort of goal—was low on the priority list of real life. After I had kids, the situation worsened, with two new little humans competing for my time and energy.

For the rest of that weekend at the tournament, I observed Sara around the rink and how happy and fit she seemed. It wasn't just that she worked out a lot; she came across as a healthy person in general, interacting with her husband and children in a way that I found inspiring. Sunday morning at breakfast, I overheard Sara and her husband negotiating when each of them was going to train that day while the other handled the kids. I thought it was cool that they were both committed to their own fitness, but also supportive of the other person.

When the ice hockey tournament ended, I piled our bags into the back of the station wagon, got into the driver's seat to pull away, and noticed Sara in the parking lot. I rolled the window down and asked if I could email her for the name of her coach. While I certainly didn't have any aspirations to become a bodybuilder, Sara had mentioned that her coach also provided nutrition and exercise consulting to noncompetitive clients.

I almost forgot about the exchange, but when I came home, Sara's email with her coach's contact information was already in my inbox. Soon after that I found myself working with a coach named Brandi Adams. I told Brandi that my primary goal was to get back in shape after a tough period in my life. I just wanted to feel good when I looked in the mirror. (How hard is that, right?) As a first step, Brandi asked me to start keeping a log of what I ate, and we found that daily calories were scattered and unpredictable: some days as high as 2,600, and others as low as 880.

And even though the number on the scale seemed reasonable for my height and stature—around 123 pounds—that weight didn't reflect how bad I was feeling and how my confidence had been sapped.

My coach assigned daily weight-based workouts with exercises I worried would make me grow hair on my chest: squats, deadlifts, bench presses. I hadn't held a barbell in decades, but I now wielded one and was able to throw on more weight each week. As the weeks went by, I could see nice changes in my body. I've always put on muscle pretty easily. My siblings and I all have wiry, mesomorphic body types with broad shoulders. Now muscles reemerged in my legs and my arms, and my midsection was notably tighter. That summer, for the first time in a long time, I wore a two-piece swimsuit.

In my weightlifting sessions, I finally found a place where I fit. What I was learning, with my coach's guidance, was leading me to rethink my whole way of relating to my body and nutrition. What if instead of using exercise and food as a tool to diminish myself, I could use them to be *more* of myself? What if I could actually *increase* my strength and capacity through working out and eating more? I'd always feared carbs and fatty foods, assuming they would make me put on weight, but Brandi explained that accepting whole foods—and eating more of them—would help me build muscle while *eliminating* fat. My coach spoke to me like an athlete. At my highest point in the coming months, I would eat 2,600 calories a day.

I felt a powerful shift taking shape within me. Simply by making myself a priority, I found my confidence. I joined a gym and made new friends. I planned my day around meals and gym visits to make sure I was taking the time to eat, rest, and exercise. I made it a daily habit to step away from my desk to lift weights.

Lifting became a metaphor: In each of my lifts, I felt I was grabbing all of life's crap and imagining it on a bar that I could hoist over my head. Pushing and pulling weights was my way of powering my muscles to get through the next onslaught of whatever life threw at me. As I was getting stronger physically, I was getting stronger mentally, too.

The act of lifting weights releases dopamine—often referred to as the "happy hormone"—which transmits messages in the brain that lead to feelings of reward, satisfaction, and motivation. Dopamine helps with other body functions including sleep, memory, movement, and focus.[1] It also stimulates a rise in noradrenaline (also known as norepinephrine), which increases alertness and attention.[2]

Psychologists who study sports behavior also say that the intensity of lifting weights actually fuels a rewiring of the brain, connecting the activity to enjoyment—and wanting more of it. It's known as neuroplasticity.

What did all this feel like? My body just worked better. I slept better. I wasn't so anxious. I stopped drinking as much—not because of any moral reason, but just because I felt I didn't need to. I even pooped more regularly. The benefits of lifting weights and eating were tangible: I was myself, just a new and improved version. Getting out there and doing stuff at the gym made me feel like I could get more things done in my life. After working out, I came back to my desk feeling refreshed and creative. My work got better, and my ideas became more ambitious. As I started to learn more about this way of treating my body, I was stunned by the ways it was improving my life.

Science backs up my experience. Studies show that women in particular benefit from weight training, even more than men do. According to a study supported by the National Institutes of Health using data from four hundred thousand adults over two decades, women who participated in strength-based exercises had a 19 percent reduced risk for death compared with those who did not exercise. Women who strength trained saw an even bigger reduction in cardiovascular-related deaths.[3] This is especially significant, as heart disease is the leading cause of death for women in the United States. There are many other ways that science illuminates the power of weight training in women: reduced incidence of certain types of cancer;[4] increased metabolism; decreased risk of dementia; prevention of bone loss; and lessened chance of injury due to falls. A growing body of research shows that strength training has a strong antidepressant effect, even among those who don't suffer from clinical depression. One study, published in *Psychiatry Research,* investigated how effective an eight-week training program of one-on-one sessions consisting of squats, deadlifts, and lunges performed twice a week could affect fifty-five young people between the ages of twenty-one and thirty-one—both with and without anxiety or depression. The results were significant, "clinically-meaningful, large-magnitude reductions in depressive symptoms" among all participants.[5] Researcher Brett R. Gordon, a postdoctoral fellow at Penn State College of Medicine who helped lead the research, says that more-depressed subjects tend to benefit the most.

It turns out you don't need to overexert yourself at the gym to derive benefits from strength-training exercises. Researchers in Japan looked at data from sixteen studies published from 2012 to 2020 comparing exercise habits with various health outcomes. They found that participants who did some type of strengthening exercise for just thirty to sixty minutes a week had a 10 to 17 percent lower risk of mortality, heart disease, and cancer.[6]

My only regret when I started working out more was that I hadn't started when I was younger, but now there was no stopping me. I rearranged my schedule to do extra work at night or early in the morning before the kids woke up. Often my mother, who lives a few doors down, would watch my girls. I loved how proud my children were of me. One day while picking up my youngest daughter at her preschool, I heard her tell a friend that her mommy looked like Wonder Woman. I created a profile on Match.com and started wearing lipstick again.

My coaches began to tell me that I had potential. They encouraged me to enter a competition, even though my chicken-skinny legs needed a lot of muscle and shaping packed on. Initially, I wasn't sure about competing. I'd seen pictures and thought the fake tans were cheesy. Were those sequined thongs? It was all trashy, crayon-colored, and over-the-top fabulous. What would my mother think?

And then one day I decided not to give a shit. I told my coaches, yes, what the heck, let's do this. I signed up for a competition that would take place several months later in May. I started preparing to compete. I ran through my lifts, day in and day out, and most important, even on those days when I really didn't feel like it or was tired. There were many excuses that I could have used—the kids needed me, it was a hard day at work, it was getting late—but I made sure there was always some way to get my workout done, whether that meant getting up before my kids did or asking for help if I needed someone to watch them. That latter piece was especially important: I sucked up my pride and reached out for a hand. I prioritized myself: The house was messy; a million things needed my attention. But the work got done. Soon the muscles became part of my identity. I owned my appearance. It belonged to me, and I felt good about being a part of a community that applauded and encouraged the effort that went into it.

Bodybuilding had become a part of who I was, the answer to people's questions about my arms or my shoulders. "What do you do?" they'd ask. And instead of just saying that I worked out, I started to tell them, "I'm a bodybuilder."

Then in March 2020, the pandemic threw my routine off course. On the thirteenth, an announcement came over the loudspeaker that the gym doors would close early. I went to the locker room and kind of sat there, wondering if and when I would ever be back. I ended up taking all the stuff out of my locker just in case—water bottle, hairbrush, towels—and put it all in a box. But when I left and stepped out onto the sidewalk, I paused, turned back around, and stuffed it all back in the locker! I didn't want my journey to end this way. The following weekend, I dragged my new partner Rick to rural Virginia to buy $900 worth of used gym equipment that I set up in my basement so I could keep working out.

While everyone was locked in and locked down, staying the course proved difficult. For one thing, my May competition was canceled. And I broke my diet several times, digging into those little lunchbox treats I stashed in a cupboard.

During this period of prepping for my first competition, I found a lot of support in my Facebook group for women who trained with the same coach. These women became my friends and teammates, even though I had hardly met any of them in real life. We experienced the same plateaus and celebrated the same highs. Fridays were always the day of the week when we posted pictures of ourselves flexing with the hashtag #FlexFriday and praised one another's small victories, like a new bump in a bicep or a bigger, more developed quadricep.

I'd connected with an extraordinary community of like-minded women who considered themselves life athletes and reveled in building themselves. Contrary to everything I'd ever been taught in the past about the female form—that women should ideally be delicate, feminine, and above all as skinny as possible—they delighted in seeing their bodies getting bigger. I loved that these women were racially, religiously, politically, and economically diverse. Nancy lives in a big house with a pool and has since started her own fitness consulting business. Rolita posts about taking vacations with her new husband and finding time for their daily devotional Bible readings. Sherille is an Army officer and fitness ambassador. Nancy and Rolita are in their fifties; Sherille is in her forties. I had met a world of women whom I would never have encountered otherwise.

I learned firsthand that when women are good to one another and supportive of each other's goals, they really benefit—more so than men. Research published in the *Harvard Business Review* points out that women who have an inner circle of close female contacts are more likely to land better and more lucrative executive jobs.[7] For men, the gender composition of their inner circles didn't matter as much. In other words, women shine when they have a network of strong, supportive women.

In June, my coach asked if I would be interested in doing a competition that had opened up in August. I quickly responded yes. I pulled out the clear plastic heels I'd bought for the first contest and regularly practiced posing in front of a full-length mirror. On August 8, 2020, I drove more than three hours to Kenilworth, New Jersey, where the competition was held. I packed the girl-power workout mix my daughters loved—our quarantine soundtrack—and sang our favorite pump-up tunes on the way.

Because of the pandemic, the audience was going to be kept to fewer than twenty-five people, so my children would watch the live stream from home with my mom and their dad. Contestants were going to wear masks, even onstage, and I had one made to match my purple bikini. Driving into the parking lot, I noticed a Wild West of red state and blue state bumper stickers. Inside the hotel, I lined up with my fellow contestants to take a polygraph test sitting in a chair tied up with tubing, where we were asked whether we'd taken performance-enhancing drugs. After that, we were instructed to don dark-colored, loose pajamas to help our spray tans set better. I followed along as we went inside small tents where ladies armed with spray guns hosed us down, everyone emerging the color of Oompa-Loompas and walking around the hotel covered in sticky orange spray and wearing dark pajamas. It was like a deranged middle-aged lady's slumber party–meets–beauty pageant, complete with meltdowns, freak-outs, and fake nails. It was also about as far as I could get from the straitlaced intellectual world of the sterile newspaper office that I usually inhabited.

After the polygraph and tanning were over, I went to get changed and (the best part) got my makeup done. The vibe across dressing rooms and backstage was a good mix of competition and camaraderie. I mean, I wanted to win and to kick ass; I'd worked hard and felt I looked the business. But my competitive streak was tempered by the simple joy I found in meeting people during a shared crazy experience. I also finally got to meet in person some of the friends on my team—and we cheered one another on.

When I was done with my makeup, I took a look in the mirror, and I loved what I saw. Big hair, fake tan, long nails, curled lashes, and all the muscles. This was unabashedly mega and meta me—with no apologies. After years of being a good girl—being quiet, waiting my turn, respecting the hierarchy and order of things—flaunting a rhinestone bikini body at my age felt deliciously inappropriate. As I walked onto the surprisingly tiny stage for my first contest, I shrugged off my nerves. Here I was in public, but not as a *Wall Street Journal* reporter. I was enjoying being nothing other than Contestant No. 41. And on that stage, I could be whoever I wanted to be.

In front of a half-dozen judges, I followed orders: "Half turn to the right." "Walk to the back." "Turn around and walk to the front." I moved through a series of walks and poses I'd practiced for months in advance, perfecting my proper strut in clear stripper heels. I smiled through my mask. I performed this same routine several times that day: competing in four divisions and placing first in three, and second in my class for another. No. 41 was a winner. I felt, for the first time in my life, that my body was not only accepted in a sport but really valued.

My results earned me a pro card—the coveted qualification that allows a bodybuilder to compete as a professional. In 2022 I competed again as an amateur, winning in the master's division and coming in first in my class in the open. I trained (stupidly) even when I was sick with COVID—which led to a bout with Long COVID. I managed one competition that year and then decided to rest and get better.

Despite the setbacks, I discovered that I love competing. This realm is completely different from the newsroom. That world of book smarts was where I once placed extraordinary value and tried hard to fit in. The bodybuilding world, however, is the direct opposite. Here it doesn't matter what you know or believe or think—it's how ripped you are. Each competition is a carnival of characters from around the country arriving in trucks and Teslas, combining reunion and pageantry for mainly middle-aged men and women. (Though it's the women who steal the show.) Often the same athletes return in a cycle of about every eighteen months; you see the same coaches, and everyone has worked hard and is ready to show off new muscles on a tiny stage. In a competition, only bodies matter, regardless of whether you are Black or white, a waitress or a trophy wife. The gatherings transcend economic, class, and social status. It is the complete opposite of the parade of rake-thin models and influencers in magazines, advertising, and social media, all of whom seem to come from the same pool of privilege (whether it's real or fake).

In the four years since that first competition, I have occasionally fallen off the wagon. I get tired like everyone else. Sometimes my workouts are phoned in. Sometimes I can't make it to the gym for one reason or another. I never say no to pizza or birthday cake. It's life. But I never, ever throw in the towel. The through line in my life is that I'm an athlete. Being an athlete isn't something that's true of you when you're young and then it's over when you grow up. It's a state of mind that allows you to push through the tough stuff and carry on.

Building my body has redefined femininity for me. What does the term *feminine* mean? It is something ingrained in us through images, in stories, in fashion, and through consumer products, and it's pretty much everything I have tried to imitate and to be. In traditional femininity, we see ourselves in the way men would like to see us. We place value in "pretty," in "slim." It is who we aspire to be in the eyes of men. And as a result it has shaped how I walk in the world. But by actively building my body into something strong—a state I believe I was born to inhabit—I feel able to defend myself and take care of myself. I don't worry or fear as much. And I no longer look in the mirror to criticize myself and find mistakes. Of course my body isn't perfect as I continue to age, but those imperfections are part of the fabric, of the texture, of this home I have built for myself.

It's thanks to bodybuilding that I came to the message of this book: that we, as women, have been brainwashed our entire lives to reduce our bodies, to make ourselves less—but that we are so much more. Everything about our culture as it relates to fitness for women is about becoming skinnier. Even the words we use around exercise are couched in diet culture. A poster in front of a Pilates studio in my neighborhood advertises a class called "Burn." In other words, it's all about burning fat, not about getting strong.

Meanwhile, women's bodies are badass. We live longer than men. We bring life into the world. Research out of Cambridge University shows that prehistoric female bones were the size of world championship rowers' bones today.[8] It's only in recent generations that society has pressured women to diminish themselves, to literally waste away.

Women don't see alternatives. In sports, we don't get the coverage and unabashed hero worship available to male athletes. Although participation in sports by school-age girls increased to one in three from one in twenty-seven in the half a century since Title IX was born,[9] a 2021 study by researchers at Purdue University and the University of Southern California shows that women's athletic representation in the media is still sorely lacking. The researchers found that in 2019, coverage of women athletes on televised news and highlight shows, including ESPN's *SportsCenter*, totaled only 5.4 percent of all airtime.[10] Young girls watching television are seeing a tiny number of women athletes on TV, and so they're not being presented with alternative body ideals. Instead, they are getting the message that society doesn't value women who look strong and powerful, at least not enough to put them out there in the wider culture and media. Caitlin Clark, who revolutionized the sport of basketball by becoming the all-time leading scorer in the game's collegiate history—regardless of gender—made $76,535 in her rookie season with the Indiana Fever. (By comparison, Zaccharie Risacher, the No. 1 pick in the NBA draft that year, is expected to earn over $12.5

million in his rookie year with the Atlanta Hawks.) How is this remotely justifiable? What does this tell our daughters about how society views them?

"It's not just about role modeling," says Cheryl Cooky, a professor at Purdue University who helped lead the research and continues to collect data on mainstream coverage of women's sports. "But it's also recognizing that's what society values."

I want to change that paradigm once and for all.

My goal is to show you that fitness and wellness can and should be a way to build—rather than shrink—yourself. That you don't need to exercise as a kind of punishment anymore. This book will help you to realize all the ways you've been conditioned to think about your body and food, and all the ways you will benefit when you can imagine *so much more* for yourself.

This isn't a book to train you to be a competitive bodybuilder—I know that's not going to be for everyone—but my love for the sport informs everything I'm writing about here because bodybuilding is fundamentally about building ourselves. I actually get excited when I see muscle growth in the mirror, and this has translated into growth in my confidence and my spirit. At the same time, bodybuilding has shifted my approach to food, helping me to make choices that maximize my health, including the way I want my body to look. Carbs don't make you fat. Fat doesn't even make you fat. But eating these and other macro- and micronutrients in the right amounts in proportion to one another can carve out a body. As a result, I eat more and choose whole foods.

Even if competitive bodybuilding isn't for you, no matter your age, gender, or body shape, you can easily add strength and resistance training to your exercise routine. This can take the form of working out with weights or with resistance bands, or of using your body weight to increase strength. (As I'll explain, you won't even need very much equipment to do this.) For too long, women have been told to focus on cardio-based workouts like aerobics, walking, running, or spinning (all of which have their place in a balanced workout routine), but studies show that if you want to protect yourself from disease, injury, and even premature death, you need to add strength training to your routine and prioritize it. Somehow this message has gotten lost in our skinny-obsessed culture, and I want to shout it from the rooftops, loud and clear.

Wellness approaches for women can be coddling, coaxing us to take the easier path. The messages sent to us by advertisers and influencers are steeped in a prevailing consumer culture. Here's a cream. Take a supplement or an injection. These pants will hide your flaws. Strength and resistance training guides us toward being more dogged, determined, and driven to achieve our goals. I've included my own story in this book, as well as the stories of other women who have made strength training or bodybuilding part of their lives, to give you a road map for practicing acts of wellness, self-care, and trying to do better *without seeking perfection*. This work is hard, but it's not to be feared. Rather, the work itself *is* a form of self-care.

I want you to recognize and own your inner athlete.

You are an athlete. You have always been one. Women's lives are an athletic feat of navigating roles and persevering when life puts sticks in your wheels, whether that means caring for others, parenting, leading, or speaking up when society has told you to be quiet and demure and not to ruffle too many feathers. You have all the strength you need within yourself. Now you just need to come home to the body you were born to inhabit.

This book is divided into three parts. The first part tells the story of skinny: how we got the idea that women need to be thin above all else. It illuminates a clampdown in the late-nineteenth and twentieth centuries to keep women in a more childlike, controlled state—not in the naturally strong condition that's our birthright.

The second part of the book is about why any of this matters: how building a life of strength has extraordinary benefits for us as we age, and how you can impart that wisdom to the next generation of girls and women.

The last part of the book shows you how to conquer the mental game and how to adjust your mindset. After all, the mind is the biggest muscle you can grow. In this part of the book, I'll show you practical and actionable approaches for adjusting the way you think about food and exercise, based on my training as a pro bodybuilder.

My biggest message to you is that yes, it's possible to take your body back, to be strong, to take up space. You can find that inner cavewoman warrior and let her help you build a stronger, longer life. And if the full-on cavewoman warrior vibe isn't quite the fit, then throw in some clear stripper heels, a spray tan, and a sparkly bikini. Who says you can't have it both ways?

PART ONE

PULL

Pulling Back the Curtain on
the Story of Women's Bodies

CHAPTER 1

THE STORY OF SKINNY

How We Got the Idea We Were Supposed to Be Thin

When I was twelve years old, in the sixth grade, I loved to go to the school library to check out the magazines on display: *Teen Beat, Tiger Beat, Bop, SuperTeen*, and *Seventeen*. During the 1980s, these magazines were a pre-TikTok guide to what teenagers needed to covet and how they should look. If you remember the genre of magazines as well as I do, you probably recall an occasional poll called "Who Wore It Better?": two side-by-side pictures of female celebrities who happened to be photographed wearing the same outfit. "Who looked better?" the magazine asked its readers. I could predict the winner before looking at the editors' percentages at the bottom. The formula was easy: It was always the thinner one.

For a preadolescent girl, that recurring magazine feature neatly summarized what seemed to be an unbreakable rule: When it comes to women, the winner is always thinner.

In my teens, I became an athlete—a figure skater, then a collegiate rower—but quickly learned my physique wasn't going to be suitable for either of those sports. I wasn't small enough and nowhere near skinny enough as a skater, and I wasn't tall enough to be a rower. This was a huge loss for me because these sports provided an escape, somewhere to go away from the day-to-day, where the only thing to worry about was a movement, a skill to master, or a time to beat.

I loved skating more than anything else—the smell of cold air, the feeling of gliding. At the rink, I was in a separate universe, and the community was a refuge. I skated nearly every day, sometimes before school, sometimes after school. I did some competitions and didn't leave any great impressions. It didn't matter—I loved all of it. I watched figure skating events on television and would drink in the music, hit rewind and slow motion to fully appreciate technique performed by the masters, and try to learn, to mimic, and to be challenged. The ice rink was a place where I could flee from school and all the social pressures of being a misfit, intimidated by institutional team sports and the confounding social hierarchies. Gliding on the ice, learning and perfecting jumps and spins felt freeing, almost otherworldly. But as much as I loved this sport, my body wasn't ever quite right. I wasn't rail-thin and was awkwardly filling out, developing breasts. I didn't have that ballerina-svelte frame that the advanced girls all seemed to have.

This feeling of fundamental inadequacy in a sport I loved became clear when I was sick with mononucleosis in the winter of my sophomore year of high school. I was away from school and the rink for about a month. When I came back to the ice, a coach noticed I looked different. "Have you lost weight?" she asked. I said that maybe I had, I'd been sick for a month. "Looks good," she said, without missing a beat. It was a moment that stayed with me for a long time. In that moment of my burgeoning adulthood, the message had never been clearer: It's worth being sick to look the part.

When I moved away to college, I discovered rowing. I was intrigued by this sport because it required so much intensity, and I liked that. I had experienced that kind of focus with skating, and this was an exciting new sport to discover. I was introduced to training in order to become bigger and stronger, and weight rooms were part of my life for the first time. Here, in this sport, the athletes weren't petite ballerinas in frilly skirts. Instead, these women were big and strong and proud of it. They showed grit. They pulled oars and pressed weights. And for the first time, I was surrounded by a new female ideal: that bigger was better.

But again I came up short. The coaches prized the tallest girls, their long limbs coveted for big sweeps of the oars. They got the choicest seats in the boats. It didn't matter that I worked extra hard; I couldn't grow taller than my five-four height. At the end of that freshman season, I was demoted to the back of the boat, even though I had produced the team's best individual time on a 2,000-meter test. The message was clear as a bell in yet another sport I loved: My body wasn't right here, either. It was another way for me to miss the mark, to feel not enough.

For me, dieting began in college. Living in all-female dorms meant ceaseless discussion about what outfits we should wear, what celebrities wore, and what looked right, desirable, and appealing. The correlation was clear—if unspoken—between looking good and being thin. Hence, talk in dorm kitchens always revolved around calories, low-fat foods, nutrition labels, serving sizes, and the too-muchness and not-enoughness. I began looking at myself in the mirror in a more critical way. Fat became a point of obsession; I watched fat grams closely on food packages and my body. While athletics should have been my refuge, my *more* of me, I began to view participation as a way to reduce myself, get rid of fat, and achieve this ideal that eluded me.

After I graduated from college, the focus changed to how my body looked in society, and success also seemed to mean thinness. A casual *Those pants look good on you* uttered by a female editor in the elevator as I headed up to my desk on the ninth floor might have been meant as a warm compliment, but the unspoken subtext was that they made me look thinner. The activities available to me at this point were in class form—yoga class, cycling class—and then, of course, there were the jogging groups, the mothers pushing their strollers while running in the park. The fun of sports—people in the weight room horsing around, confident and cursing, hugging and slapping each other's butts after a surprising win—was gone from my life. Exercise classes were carefully branded with names like "Lengthen" and "Burn," with a nod to burning calories to get thinner, or if muscle was mentioned, it was "lean" muscle to "tone" just a bit. Another way to feel not enough.

Although we've made such strides in how we represent and elevate races, genders, and sexual orientations, mainstream society's preoccupation with female thinness is just as pervasive to me now as it was when I was in sixth grade. Reminders of skinniness—how to seek it, where to find it, how we are not enough because of it—are the drumbeat of a woman's day-to-day existence. After a while, you even stop noticing the constancy of it, sort of like the color of paint on the walls around you. It's in the name of the brand of crackers and popcorn we buy and the cut of jeans we wear. A package of Uncle Vinny's Romaine lettuce implores consumers to "stay skinny with Uncle Vinny." The company Skinnygirl—which reality star Bethenny Frankel sold to the company that makes Jim Beam for a reported $100 million[1]—offers reduced-calorie cocktails and wines and urges women to "drink like a lady." Froneri's Skinny Cow brand pitches ice cream as diet food to women. The list goes on, from Skinnypop to Lean Cuisine.

From the time a mother tugs "skinnies" over her baby girl's diaper, women are conditioned to associate thinness with pleasing others and enjoying feelings of love and acceptance. This "ideal" is baked into our very brains. Skinny is the privileged vessel that rises above all others—the chosen one—and anything else seems an affront. Women with strong, powerful, and well-nourished bodies are rarely represented in advertisements or championed on the screen. "You have to be thin," says a frustrated Gloria, played by America Ferrera, in the 2023 summer blockbuster movie *Barbie*. "But not too thin. And you can never say you want to be thin. You have to say you want to be healthy, but also you have to be thin."[2]

When I ran into thirty-four-year-old Sara, the bodybuilder, in a hotel gym, she was sweaty, red-faced, and focused, recording her results in an app. Her physique wasn't skinny. Instead, it was built through hard work, the muscles clear, defined, and power-ful. Later I returned to my room and looked hard at myself in the mirror. *What had happened?* I'd spent the last two decades of my life critiquing myself in the mirror, on various diets, cutting carbohydrates—always disappointed, obsessed with trying to get numbers on the scale to go down. What if I had been focus-ing on the wrong thing?

As I began to train with weights and gained more confidence in my body—taking pride in my newfound muscles—I realized it felt good to shed not so much the pounds, but the whole idea of skinny.

This body I now inhabited vastly differed from the version I had sought my whole life. Being a strong woman was a profound homecoming—I felt happy, comfortable, and *sound*. I ate well and I ate a lot, enjoying my food and the feeling of nourishment and strength it offered to me. Which was why it was such a shock to the system when, as I began prepping to compete for the first time as a bodybuilder, I learned I was going to have a short period of restricting calories immediately before the contest in order to cut—aka look spectacular in a bikini. My coach, Tina, explained that although for most of our training, bodybuilders put the focus on eating plentifully and growing muscle, we cut back on the calories immediately before the event so that our muscles can be fully visible to the judges.

While I was cutting, the change in my mood was marked. To put it simply, I felt downright cranky most of the time, and I couldn't wait to eat fully again once the competition was over. After competing, I was immensely relieved to return to my usual calorie intake. I felt human again. "We tell our athletes over and over again that they can cut weight, but over the long term, that is not sustainable," Tina reassured me. "A muscular body cannot stay muscular on a calorie deficit."

This experience of restricting calories not only led me to value eating well (that is, a plentiful intake of nutrient-rich food) but also prompted me to reflect. How did we get here? Why are women expected to be skinny, even when competing in a sport that's about strength and power? Why do we spend so much time, money, energy, and brainpower trying to be thinner when that means literally diminishing ourselves? As I began reading about the feminine physique and the ways in which expectations have shifted over the course of history, I learned that we haven't always wanted to look like twigs.

In fact, the glorification of female skinniness is a construct of control, the product of the last hundred years of history that gets more extreme, impossible, unsustainable, and dangerous as time goes on, an ideal we've bought into without thoroughly questioning how it serves us.

Graham Crackers and Gibson Girls

You don't have to look very far back to find a time *before* we were obsessed with skinny. Not so long ago, women actually wanted to be bigger.

In the eighteenth and nineteenth centuries, agricultural innovations—most notably crop rotation, which resulted in better soil and more significant livestock and crop yields—led to a substantial increase in food supply.[3] For centuries, plumpness had been a sign of wealth—the ability to afford ample food. In those days, having enough to eat separated the haves from the have-nots; it was a status symbol, and there was no hiding who had access to the stuff. During a time when malnutrition was still a threat, more flesh on the body was considered a good thing—an ideal that was reflected in arts, literature, and medical opinion alike.[4] Wealth helped inform the standard of beauty back then,[5] and by the time the 1870s rolled around, well-to-do women were even adding padding to their frames, emphasizing curvy bottoms and hips with bustles. The richer the woman, the bigger her voluminous behind.

In the 1870 book *Personal Beauty: How to Cultivate and Preserve It in Accordance with the Laws of Health,* American doctors Daniel Garrison Brinton and George Henry Napheys wrote in praise of big women, pointing out that a "scrawny bony figure" is "intolerable to gods and men." In fact, they explained, feminine thinness could only possibly come in handy if someone were trying to deter a cannibal.[6]

But this golden era when physicians like Brinton praised bigger women for their health and vitality was not to last. A burgeoning movement against "corpulence" was already under way.

A Presbyterian minister named Sylvester Graham had begun making waves in New England for his sermons equating morality and temperance with abstinence from all kinds of yum, including meat, spices, alcohol, and tobacco. Sex more than once a month was depravity. In particular, his support for vegetarianism and criticism of refined flour drew the most attention.

After experimenting with coarsely ground wheat, Graham created graham flour, followed by graham bread and eventually the graham cracker in 1829.[7] He railed against commercial white bread, which was being mass-produced thanks to industrialization, a sign of modern times. In his *Treatise on Bread, and Bread-Making,* Graham wrote: "Thousands in civic life will, for years, and perhaps as long as they live, eat the most miserable trash that can be imagined in the form of bread, and never seem to think that they can possibly have anything better, not even that it is an evil to eat such vile stuff as they do."[8]

Sylvester Graham believed that gluttony was the result of civilization and refinement. He linked the virtues of womanhood, particularly motherhood, with cooking and baking with the purest and most simple ingredients.

Graham's theory of diet was also a theory of femininity and social order, borne of whole ingredients that didn't whet appetites into too much of a tizzy and raised children who could withstand the vileness of modernity. His acolytes were the first Weight Watchers. They lived on a diet of fresh fruits and vegetables, wheat bread, rice, and a bit of cream. They took pride in eating slowly, taking meals six hours apart, and avoiding snacking. The letters and testimonials of Grahamites indicate the first evidence of ordinary Americans who regularly weighed themselves.[9]

Graham's influence reached across the Atlantic. In England, an undertaker named William Banting followed a diet that helped him shed around fifty pounds from his 202-pound frame, which inspired him to write a pamphlet called *Letter on Corpulence* in 1863, which he addressed to the public. The strict low-carbohydrate diet was prescribed by a doctor who instructed him to give up foods that contained starch and sugars, such as bread, butter, milk, sugar, beer, and potatoes. The pamphlet was popular for years, was reprinted multiple times, and was cited by physicians and cooking schools, including in the United States. It is widely regarded as a progenitor of popular modern low-carb diets. In some cultures, *banting* is synonymous with dieting. In Swedish, *banta* is a verb for slimming down.

In 1899, an American insurance examiner named George R. Shepherd, president of the Association of Life Insurance Medical Directors of America, lamented the absence of statistics on obesity. Shepherd looked at preliminary data from several insurance companies, which suggested that "from our mortality records the overweights are clearly less desirable than either the normal or the underweights."[10]

The American war on weight had officially begun. By now, a new feminine ideal was already taking shape in the form of hugely popular magazine illustrations by the American illustrator Charles Dana Gibson. Gibson began publishing pen-and-ink sketches of his "Gibson girls" in *Life* and other magazines starting in the 1890s.[11] Gibson's modern women were beautiful and confident. They sometimes stared down at the viewer instead of casting their eyes aside modestly, as so many women subjects had done before. The Gibson girl was talented—she could sing, draw, and play the violin while looking youthful and stylish. She was often depicted engaging in physical, playful activities such as bicycling and playing tennis. Even though corsets were still around to help squeeze her into an hourglass shape,[12] the Gibson girl's body was noticeably longer and leaner. A new ideal was emerging. All of a sudden, women were being fed the idea that they should aspire to be slim.

Gibson's pen-and-ink drawings, Graham's disciples, and Banting's testimonial all came at a time when the role of women in society was expanding rapidly. These post–Industrial Revolution bros were agents of a patriarchy that gaslit women into minimizing themselves. This was an attempt at control, a scramble to weaken women as they gained influence and disrupted the social order. The women's suffrage movement was well on its way, doggedly inching toward its goal of enfranchising women. The New Woman was independent, educated, and youthful, and she embraced a more prominent public role.[13] She was infiltrating college campuses and professional arenas at a startling pace. Slowly, men's control over the opposite sex was dwindling.

Is it any coincidence that the pressure to be thin coincided with a newly empowered woman who wanted political agency? As the American author and feminist Naomi Wolf wryly noted in her seminal 1991 book *The Beauty Myth,* "soft, rounded hips and thighs and bellies were perceived as desirable and sensual without question until women got the vote."[14] In one study, authors Brett Silverstein and Deborah Perlick tracked the curvaceousness of *Vogue* cover models with female college graduation rates over several decades, finding that increases in the proportion of women graduating from college correlated to a slimmer standard, an indication that a less curvaceous physique translated to more professional opportunity.[15]

One early victim of the new trend for slimming down was the singer and actress Lillian Russell. Russell was a curvy star whom *The Saturday Evening Post* described in the 1890s as "a voluptuous beauty and there was plenty of her to see. We liked that. Our tastes were not thin or ethereal. We liked flesh in the nineties."[16] Russell, who sang in theater, was considered beautiful even as she neared 200 pounds.[17] Once described as "the raging beauty of her period," she was selected to make the first public long-distance telephone call by singing to President Grover Cleveland at the White House. (Take that, Marilyn Monroe.)[18] Her constant companion was James Buchanan "Diamond Jim" Brady, an American businessman and financier, who was reputed to have a legendary appetite.[19] The two were frequently seen dining together; she is said to have enjoyed food just as much as he did. It was considered part of her sex appeal.

But times were changing, and Russell was forced to change her habits. The press now criticized Russell for her figure, with a reporter for the *New York Journal* even writing that "Lillian has no beauty below the chin."[20] Russell took such criticisms to heart. Diamond Jim got her a bicycle, plated with gold and encrusted with gemstones. Before long, she became the poster child for the new fad of "reducing," which, for Lillian, involved riding that bicycle all over New York City to shed weight. In an 1896 article, a reporter spotted her and wrote: "Miss Russell went for her usual ride in Central Park yesterday afternoon. She wore a tan bicycle suit that fitted as if she had been melted and run into it."[21]

Russell gave interviews on her various other weight-loss attempts, which included rolling over 250 times in the morning. She exercised with barbells and punching bags, but she never managed to whittle her physique down to this impossible new ideal, and how could she? By the 1920s, "slimness, leanness and flatness are the order of the day . . . the figures of our flappers and subdebs shall be slender and slinky and lathlike and the line of grace no longer the curve but the prolonged parallelogram," according to a writer in *The Saturday Evening Post*.[22] Russell's struggles with weight likely paved the way to her decline. Her voice deteriorated, and her last appearances were in vaudeville until she retired in 1919, only a year before white women finally won the right to cast a ballot in this country.

Before dieting entered the picture, this woman had been in her prime: performing, feasting, serving as an object of desire. Did society's pressure to box her in coincide with or cause her voicelessness?

Enter the Gamine

As women entered the 1920s, a thin frame became all the rage. At this point, fashionable women were flappers; they smoked cigarettes, drove cars, danced, and wore bold lipstick. Shorter hemlines replaced big hoop skirts. Stiff corsets and bodices gave way to foundation undergarments that allowed more movement. New brassieres contained materials, such as elastic, that offered movement but also flattened the chest. Even corset forms changed, de-emphasizing the waist into a more boy-like figure. The women who wore these garments were modern and revolutionary. And yet this new rake-thin figure was an odd contrast to women's increasingly muscular voices. Even Black women, who would not win the right to vote in this country until the Voting Rights Act in 1965, were also exposed to the skinny-is-beautiful imagery. The women of the Harlem Renaissance—a cultural revival of Black music and art taking place in New York City's Harlem in the 1920s—often embodied the look of the gamine. Its heroines included Josephine Baker, her long limbs set off by sleeveless dresses, and Billie Holiday, often emaciated from her addiction to heroin.

Of all the weight-loss evangelists of the new century, Lulu Hunt Peters was one of the most significant influences on American women. Peters was an American physician who wrote a syndicated column called "Diet and Health," which ran in some four hundred newspapers in the early twentieth century.[23] Peters, who weighed over 200 pounds at one point, began following her own health regimens, and readers loved her. Her columns led to a book, published in 1918, called *Diet and Health: With Key to the Calories,* which laid the framework for what we know as the modern diet-book genre.

Calories were such a novel concept that Peters had to explain to readers how to pronounce the word. Writing during World War I, she called it "a crime to hoard food," adding that "there are hundreds of thousands of individuals all over America who are hoarding food. . . . They have vast amounts of this valuable commodity stored away in their own anatomy."

Peters's book sold over two million copies in the years that followed. According to *Publishers Weekly,* it was the number four bestselling nonfiction book in 1923 and laid the foundation for years of female self-torture. "Personally, I wish every time I ate a chocolate," she wrote, "I would get a worm."

Magazines and newspapers continued to publish images of idealized featherweight women. According to one study, between 1901 and 1925, the bust-to-waist ratios among women featured in America's magazines decreased by about 60 percent.

The study's authors wrote: "Such findings would constitute empirical support for the hypothesis that the mass media play a role in promoting the slim standard."[24]

In the course of a few short decades, America had gone from a country where women took pride in their curves to one where eating disorders became a new and dangerous norm. Being skinny was now a status symbol, a mark of wealth and success, and an indication that one had enough time and discipline to shed the pounds.

Grapefruits, Cigarettes, and Rainbow Pills

And so came the parade of diets, each more misery-inducing than the one before it. The Hollywood diet of the 1930s called for eating a grapefruit with every meal. Then came the cabbage diet of the 1950s, which involved eating cabbage soup around the clock. Cigarette companies tucked dieting pamphlets inside cigarette boxes. Advertisements featuring women encouraged them to "Reach for a Lucky Instead of a Sweet."[25]

Soon enough, women were reaching for pills as well. Weight-loss drugs ran the gamut, from an industrial chemical used in munitions that in 1933 was discovered to aid in weight loss to amphetamine cocktails; from rainbow diet pills in the 1950s to black beauties in the 1960s, the drugs got progressively more dangerous and addictive. Women were dying to be thin.

In the late 1960s, the British fashion model Twiggy led the way for a fashion industry that hired progressively thinner models who became household names. Of course, fashion significantly contributed to the new skinny ideal: After all, clothes were the gift wrap for how women wanted to present themselves, the vessel for thinness to be marketed and sold. The development of U.S. standard clothing sizes paved the way for women to start comparing themselves to one another, for one number to identify their self-worth and another to become a goalpost. The numbers used for sizes began to decrease to assuage women, because a smaller number meant a happier consumer. In 1958, a 34-inch bust and a 25-inch waist was a size 12. But today, a size 12 fits a 39-inch bust and a 32-inch waist.[26] And while Marilyn Monroe might have been a 12 in her day, her measurements would be closer to a 6 by today's standards.[27] "Vanity sizing" helped customers feel better about their size.

One notable study published in 1980 analyzed key metrics to illustrate this shift in body ideals for women. By using the reported weight and measurements of Miss America contestants and *Playboy* centerfolds, researchers showed these women became demonstrably thinner from 1959 to 1978. Not insignificantly, the data showed that pageant winners were typically thinner than even the average contestant, pointing to thinness as the winning standard. The study also measured the frequency of articles about dieting in six popular women's magazines, showing that the number of articles about the subject had roughly doubled in about twenty years. Wrote the authors of the study: "It is ironic that the current symbols of 'sexual attractiveness' may be gravitating toward a weight which is in biological opposition to normal reproductive activity."[28]

All About That Base

At the turn of the twenty-first century, we started to see signs of hope that the body ideal was shifting from thinness into something more relatable. In 2004, the Dove Campaign for Real Beauty aimed to address women's poor self-image. The company shifted its ad strategy from product-focused to one whose point of view came from the consumer's self-perception. The campaign featured "real women" in bare skin and underwear—rather than models—with slogans such as "tested on real curves." With these ads, Dove tried to contend with the pervasiveness of the skinny ideal. Its advertisement called "Daughters," which aired during the Super Bowl in 2006, showed images of little girls and spoke to their insecurities. "I think my thighs are fat," said one subject. "I feel pressure like that a lot and then I go home and do sit-ups," said another.

Of course, the ad helped make profits for the parent company, Unilever. The campaign increased sales from $2 billion to $4 billion in its first few years.[29] There was also criticism that while Unilever was promoting a healthier view of beauty, the other brands in the portfolio of the personal health conglomerate were still capitalizing on sexualized portrayals of women, such as Axe body spray's ads that promised an "axe effect" of making women swoon.

The Dove campaign wasn't as much of a complete turnaround as a drop in the ocean. The era of social media had arrived, and before long, we were glued to our small screens, fixated on yet more images of women—a new breed of so-called beauty and wellness influencers whose role was to sell us a concept of health tied to beauty, fitness, and exercise and the countless products associated with them. Concurrently, fitness and health magazines continued to churn out images and articles with a constant focus on weight loss. Thinness was equated with not only beauty but also healthiness.

A 2015 analysis compared captions and images of cover models in *Men's Health* and *Women's Health* magazines. It found that *Women's Health*'s displays of weight loss, dieting, and appearance-based themes encouraged women to achieve thinness, whereas the messages for men focused more on building muscularity. Men in *Men's Health* were also nearly twice as likely to be fully clothed; women were more than four times more likely to be partially clothed than men.[30]

Still, the Dove campaign made a business case for other companies to convince women that their bodies were okay and that they could buy their creams and bras without feeling like they were trying to be someone else. Advertising for American Eagle Outfitters' Aerie brand of underwear and athleisure included curvier models. The company's #AerieREAL campaign launched in 2014 with a promise to not touch up photos. A 2018 Times Square billboard proclaimed, "No Retouching on These Girls."

For some further respite from the pervasive skinny, at least in the 2010s, we could turn to hip-hop culture to see women taking up room and showcasing big, unapologetic bodies and voices, with Black women pointing the way to a larger, curvier female aesthetic. Hip-hop artist Rihanna's Savage X Fenty underwear brand has made waves with its inclusive fashion shows filled with big, bold bodies, the anti–Victoria's Secret. Beyoncé's *Lemonade* album, in which she reacted to her husband's infidelity, was a moment of true empowerment, reaching deep into the Black female experience and exploring the impacts of enslavement on the Black family, with its creator in all her full-figured glory. In the song "Juice," Lizzo, her plus-size frame enveloped in feathers and unitards, sang that she wasn't a snack but rather "the whole damn meal." And they were joined by an entire generation of female music artists who felt proud that they finally didn't have to diet down their voices or bodies. Rear ends became a look-here symbol of ownership of your image and identity. Meghan Trainor sang an anthem to big booties that was "All About That Bass." Fascination with Kim Kardashian's butt not only led to more follows on Instagram but also bolstered the financial empire of the entire family.

Before long, butts surpassed abdomens as the latest fitness craze: Gyms, from Bünda (Portuguese for "butt") to the Glute Lab in San Diego, now specialize in helping women develop a bigger bottom. Bodybuilding coaches with female athletes typically focus on "building the glutes" more than any other body part. The Brazilian butt lift, or BBL, became one of the hottest plastic surgery procedures. Was it a move toward body positivity or just another disordered obsession with a body part?

Such big-butt mania sprang up as an antidote to a new generation of Instagram influencers who were, inevitably, perfectly gorgeous and thin. Proponents of body positivity wanted to liberate women from the skinny obsession, urging us to happily occupy our bodies of all shapes, sizes, and abilities. For a while, it looked like retailers and advertisers would follow suit. In 2018, Loft and Madewell introduced plus sizes. *Sports Illustrated* started introducing plus-size models in its swimsuit edition. Old Navy introduced a Bodequality campaign that merged the retailer's women's plus-size section with regular sizes and photographed models in sizes 4, 12, and 18. It also trained store employees to communicate about size in ways that built confidence and self-esteem. "Welcome to the revolution," wrote chief executive Nancy Green, heralding the new campaign.

But something about this reassurance didn't sit well with women who had been fed quite the opposite from these companies their entire lives. In 2022, Victoria's Secret launched a mea culpa ad trying to distance itself from its "angels"—the long-standing fashion shows where for more than two decades, six-foot models with blinged-out boobs wearing wings had paraded in front of a gawking audience. After CEO Martin Waters declared the angels no longer "culturally relevant," the new ads heralded different body shapes and blunt apologies, like "we've changed" and "we see you." The ads rang false for many women, and the company pulled them. Sales of Victoria's Secret products tanked in 2023 to around $6 billion from 2020's $7.5 billion.[31] At the time of writing, the company is still trying to figure out a path forward. "Sexiness can be inclusive," said Greg Unis, a brand president, to investors. Still, hedging its bets, it brought back former models such as Naomi Campbell and Gisele Bündchen in 2023 to promote a new "Icon" collection. The company has also since said it will relaunch its fashion with a more body-inclusive spirit.

"We've read the comments and heard you," the company wrote in an Instagram post.

On August 15, 2023, the company shared its "brand values" in a post, with an explanation that it has "moved from promoting an exclusionary view of what's sexy, to celebrating all women throughout every phase of their lives."

Victoria's Secret's confusing back-and-forth shows how deeply the skinny ideal runs and that it takes more than just a couple of ad campaigns to shift our thinking. Many of these brands' efforts toward body size and shape inclusivity shut down as quickly as they started. Old Navy ended its Bodequality campaign just a year after it began when sales plummeted. Other retailers that pulled back on plus-size offerings included M.M.LaFleur; founder Sarah LaFleur wrote in an email to customers that "we've been struggling to sell enough of our plus-size clothing to offset the cost of producing it."[32] After only three years, Loft quietly ended its 2018 foray into extended plus sizes.

Yet the vast majority of American women are plus size, with two-thirds of us wearing a size 14 or larger.[33] And these women need to buy clothes! The market exists. So what's going on here? "People would rather lose out on money than have fat people wear their clothes," surmises Sarah Dealy, a writer in Los Angeles speaking on a podcast about the plus-size experience called *Weight For It*. Finding clothes appropriate to wear—whether it's to church, a party, a gym, or an office—means being able to enter and access those spaces, Dealy says. If you can't find something to wear to the party, you won't go. Not making clothes available is society's way of saying overweight people aren't welcome.

Just as Old Navy and others were shutting down their plus-size campaigns, our tortured relationship with our bodies took another turn. A new generation of weight-loss drugs hit the market. Ozempic was approved in 2017 as a treatment for diabetes but with a remarkable side effect of weight loss. While the drug was not explicitly approved for weight loss, physicians began prescribing it off-label for that use, causing shortages for those who genuinely needed it for diabetes. At a time when 40 percent of Americans are considered obese, it became so popular that four years later drug maker Novo Nordisk came out with a higher-dose version of the drug, under the name Wegovy, that was FDA-approved for weight loss. This class of diet drugs, known as semaglutides, encompassed a new category of medicine for type 2 diabetes that, unlike insulin, also helped people lose weight. (Insulin often has the reverse effect, causing weight gain.) Eli Lilly received approval for its version, called Mounjaro, in 2022. One clinical trial showed that the active ingredient in Mounjaro helped overweight participants shed at least a quarter of their body weight.[34] Eli Lilly received approval to market the drug for weight loss in 2023 under the name Zepbound.

Is Ozempic Right for Me?

Predictably, tabloids declared that thin was back with a vengeance. Headlines now screamed, "The Cult of Thinness Is Making a Depressing Comeback" and "Is Fashion Making a Worrying Return to Size Zero?" The drugs became the subject of hushed chatter at hair salons and cocktail parties about which celebrities take it and how well it works. Host Jimmy Kimmel quipped at the 95th Annual Academy Awards, "Everybody looks so great. When I look around this room, I can't help but wonder, 'Is Ozempic right for me?'"[35]

The public and the paparazzi speculated whether Kim Kardashian had used the drugs to fit into a famous Marilyn Monroe dress (which she instead attributed to diet, exercise, and drinking plenty of water).[36] When asked how he lost thirty pounds, Elon Musk tweeted that he had used "Ozempic/Wegovy." Amy Schumer said when she tried Ozempic, it made her feel sick, and she discontinued it. But she also said that she invested in the pharmaceutical company because it was obvious that these drugs were taking off like wildfire in Hollywood.[37]

Singer-songwriter Adele lost one hundred pounds in two years, dividing fans, many of whom saw themselves represented in the megastar. She said she lost the weight by embracing strength-based exercise after her divorce. In conversation with Oprah, she responded to critics of her weight loss, saying, "I feel bad it's made anyone feel horrible about themselves. It's not my job to validate how people feel about their bodies."[38]

Oprah herself, meanwhile, told *People* magazine in 2023 that thoughts about her weight "occupied five decades of space in my brain, yo-yo-ing and feeling like why can't I just conquer this thing, believing willpower was my failing" in a coming-out article that revealed that she was taking one of the new prescription weight-loss drugs.[39] Even Weight Watchers, which once benefited from having Ms. Winfrey as a spokeswoman, investor, and board member, has introduced a new program that offers the latest anti-obesity meds.

And as the masses continue to pander to celebrities as models of what they aspire to look like, the playing field just got exponentially wider. Looking like a magazine cover is just an injection away for those who can afford it—these drugs may not be covered by insurance and can cost in the region of $1,000 a month—and far less attainable for everyone else. In other words, we are comfortable calling ourselves feminists and taking up space in the boardroom and the corner office, but we are not comfortable taking up *actual* space. The calculation women make—that thin equals successful—is not without basis. One 2011 study from the Federal Reserve Bank of St. Louis that examined men's and women's wages relative to their weight showed that women who were heavier tended to earn less. The results for men, however, were more ambiguous, with some studies even showing that men considered overweight earned more.[40]

And the ideal gets ever more impossible. Now, newer research shows a growing popularity of a skinny-muscular physique. In a 2017 study, a panel of seventy-eight undergraduate students at Missouri State University analyzed images of Miss USA pageant winners from 1999 to 2013.[41] The panel of women ages eighteen to thirty-one found that the bodies became thinner and more muscular over time and therefore were rated more attractive. In a second study, researchers Brooke Whisenhunt and Frances Bozsik took about a half-dozen images from social media of thin models and then photoshopped more muscularity into the photos. The panel of sixty-four undergraduates said they found the before-and-after images equally attractive but chose the more muscular physique when prompted for their preference.[42]

So the upshot is that now, not only is it desirable to be skinny, but you also have to layer musculature onto the thinness. "It's particularly insidious because it is promoted under the guise of 'health,'" says Dr. Whisenhunt. "It's our diet and exercise market. There is money to be made, if you do these things in order to look like this."

It's also completely unrealistic. Any bodybuilding coach will tell you that while that level of leanness and muscularity is possible, it is not sustainable. Athletes enter bodybuilding competitions knowing they are presenting a "stage lean" body—achieved by a strict dieting and workout regimen—and cannot wait to start eating and lifting heavy weights again. You need plenty of calories to build muscle—a surplus of calories, in fact. A bodybuilding show is a snapshot moment in a much longer journey, a long-term period of building and getting strong. Bodybuilders cut to showcase muscle, but that ripped, lean look is not sustainable over time. Without sufficient calories, your muscles simply won't grow, no matter how much you work out.

In other words, this total dominance of thin is a kind of collective madness. And losing too much too fast can have ghastly side effects, from gallstones to the loss of precious good muscle mass that's hard to gain back as we age. Somehow we've all bought into this idea that women need to remain in their role as the "weaker sex" and that we need to forcibly fit ourselves into bodies that are smaller, thinner, and less substantial. Why? Do we instinctively sense that men need to feel better about themselves? Is there some primitive cycle of propagation at work here? Men who feel strong and good about themselves fight for and make babies with women they are attracted to and can dominate—who then reproduce and carry on lineages? In an age where women support themselves—we *can* buy ourselves flowers—are we still subscribing to this concept of beauty, a construct of control that no longer serves us and seems to get only more extreme? More important, what can we do to free ourselves from the delusion that we need to be thinner to lead lives that are fuller—in every sense of the word?

CHAPTER 2

SHE'S A BRICK HOUSE

The Original Badass Physique

After running into Sara at the hotel, I hoped to reach out to her coach, not because I was interested in becoming a bodybuilder but because I wanted to understand better what I should be eating and how I should be exercising. I wanted to work with someone who could put me on some kind of path.

"Who do you want to look like?" coach Brandi Adams asked me in February 2019. She was asking about my goals for my physique. I was stumped. I knew I wasn't supposed to point to the Kaia Gerber–type model with the thin arms, but I didn't have much else to go on. That body type had always been my reference point.

At that point, I had begun jogging and taking classes at Orangetheory, so at 123 pounds I looked fine by standards based on societal norms. However, the weights I used in the exercise classes appealed to me more than the cardio machines.

Soon after meeting Brandi, I joined the Facebook group of fitness enthusiasts and saw that on Fridays, they'd post pictures of themselves flexing their muscles with the hashtag #FlexFriday. These women didn't look perfect. They didn't even mind some extra fat in the middle. But they seemed optimistic and hardworking. They would cheer one another on. "Look at them guns!" wrote one. "Girl, you are #goals!" wrote another. I initially thought this was weird. On the other hand, the women seemed fun, approachable, and healthy. They shared recipes, small victories, struggles, and selfies. Eventually, I was drawn to participate.

After a couple of months, I started posting my own pictures, felt encouraged, and I can honestly say that's where something happened. My ideal shifted. I went from seeing skinny bodies everywhere to surrounding myself with athletic ones, where you could see the work, the diligence, the lifestyle that had gone into creating the physique. The power, grooves, and muscle became far more interesting than just a flat board. This kind of amped-up physique was something to be respected and admired and worked toward. I was also drawn to the lifestyle, the commitment to oneself, and the discipline required. I felt a well of support from women I had never met in real life—cool women who were confident and kind and encouraging to one another, and who posted supportive comments daily in this closed Facebook group.

In August 2019, I was visiting my brother in San Diego and entered a gym. A sign on the wall read, "Change Your Life." It was a cheesy commercial gym poster, but I reflected on that. I posted a picture and wrote to these new teammates: "I found you guys, and my life was forever changed."

I was now routinely following my coach's program of weight-based workouts. I did these four or five times a week, exercises that I had long associated with football players: squats, deadlifts, and bench presses. I wielded a barbell and could increase weight each week. As time passed, I loved seeing what was happening to my body. My midsection got leaner. My arms—especially my shoulders—grew in muscularity. My quadriceps were visible. In the mirror, I started seeing the outlines of the athlete I once knew.

All this went against every worry in the back of my mind: Don't lift too much weight or get too bulky. Avoid carbs. Do nothing but cardio. I wasn't aiming for weight loss now but to build muscle while eliminating fat. My coach said eating more—not less—would help feed my muscles.

After I discovered lifting, I felt like my physical self found its natural state. I was no longer working against my body but working with it—quite literally building upon it. When I feel my best, I weigh around 120 pounds and have 16 to 18 percent body fat on my five-four frame. I look fit, but not all muscle striations are visible because they are protected with a healthy layer of fat. I lift on most days and enjoy feeling satiated with carbs, greens, and homemade proteins during the week. I indulge in wine on most weekends, eat the birthday cake with my kids, and have pizza on Friday night with them. In other words, I am pretty careful with food—I do most of my own cooking and track to ensure I'm getting enough protein—but I'm not restrictive. This is the time in bodybuilding when the work happens. We call it the growth season, because muscles grow when bodies are well-fed and nourished.

My weightlifting practice synthesized how powerful I felt. The combination of adrenaline, testosterone, and endorphins made me feel like I could conquer anything. My first set would always be pathetic as I begrudgingly began the exercise. I threw a couple more plates onto the bar for the second set and gained confidence. By the third set, I could feel a burst of positive energy. I felt strong, my muscles engorged, accentuated. In a gym mirror, I would preen.

After the weightlifting repetitions, I let go of the bar, allowing it to fall to the floor with a satisfying crash. Bodybuilders have a term for this; they call it the pump. Arnold Schwarzenegger once famously compared it to sex in the 1977 film *Pumping Iron*. Turns out women kind of like it, too. Over time, I began to recognize that the body ideal I had aspired to my entire life ignored something fundamental about the way women's bodies are built.

Lessons from the Hunter-Gatherers

Today a new generation of (primarily female) academics, scientists, historians, and researchers has finally deconstructed the myth that women have always been "weaker." Take, for example, Alison Murray, an anthropology professor at the University of Victoria in Canada, who was studying prehistoric human remains when she made a startling discovery about women's bodies: They were buff.

Since anthropologists began studying our ancestors' remains, male bones have been the default ones used. Male skeletons are bigger and easier to study because they show a neatly distinguishable timeline that clarifies the role of technology in human evolution: As humans benefited from better tools, bone size and strength declined with time.

Women's bones, by comparison, showed a less clear progression, so researchers tended to ignore them. Women were considered small men and therefore less interesting. But after Alison Murray submitted a paper that tracked leg bone strength in male and female farmers in 2017, she realized maybe she was missing something important by comparing men to women.[1] Why not use a scanner in the lab to take CT scans of modern female undergraduates and compare *those* bones to the prehistoric women's ones? She scanned the leg and arm bones of eighty-two Cambridge undergraduates—a mix of nonathletes, rowers, soccer players, and runners. The rowers—with their highly developed upper bodies—showed bone structure most similar to the early women. Both groups of women had in common evidence of consistent, repetitive load-bearing activity; this also revealed that the women were at least as much a part of the development of agriculture as men.

For Murray, this completely changed the picture of early women's role in society. These prehistoric women were quite literally pulling their weight, not just out picking berries in the field. "They were killing it," Murray says.

Yet our present-day society glorifies female bodies that are underweight and malnourished. Why? Is it because the skinny physique fits the narrative of the male hunter-gatherer and his stay-at-home-in-the-cave woman? Does it come down to the yin to the yang, the strong to the weak, the man on the mission for the woman who needs protection? Certainly, the iconography of the male hunter-gatherer is pervasive; it's in storybooks and cartoons, the burly caveman wielding a club, his mate stylishly trim and wearing pearls: Wilma Flintstone as handmaiden to Fred.

Thankfully, a growing body of research completely upends that comfortable conceit that men were the ones killing animals for meat and skins while women gathered food in the fields and tended to their children.[2] The highly gendered hunter-gatherer narrative has come under scrutiny in recent times, with more and more evidence to show that women have always been strong and capable—active participants in so-called men's work. The problem is that centuries of mythmaking and folklore around women's roles have completely obscured this reality.

In 2023, anthropology professors Cara Ocobock and Sarah Lacy published a groundbreaking paper that examined the female as a hunter in Paleolithic societies.[3] The two women looked at the division of labor between men and women in prehistory to see what they could discern about the sexes and their differing roles. What they came to understand was that there was zero evidence to support the theory that men were the only ones doing the hunting. These prehistoric women were demonstrably strong and capable of participating in the physical exertions of the hunt. In light of these discoveries, Ocobock and Lacy looked into the origins of the myth of the exclusively male hunter-gatherer. They discovered it dated back to the 1960s, when a group of mostly male researchers presented a collection of "Man the Hunter" papers at a symposium on hunter-gatherer societies to great fanfare. The research pretty much ignored any evidence—which existed even then—of women's role in the hunt. That's because the researchers superimposed their twentieth-century assumptions about men's and women's roles on the story of who brought home the bacon.

A paper published in late 2023 further upends this paradigm. Researchers from Seattle Pacific University looked at cultural studies from the past 120 years illustrating sixty-three foraging societies with thousands of years of history.[4] The data indicated that 79 percent of the societies who hunted showed evidence of women hunting. For these women, hunting was an established role for females within the social structure, not just something they did now and again to pinch-hit for the men. The study showed that women even had their own style of hunting. In certain cases, while men typically clung to one tool, women were more fluid about how they hunted, apparently switching capably from one tool to another depending on the context. Women also taught their children to hunt. Among the indigenous Agta people of the Philippines, for instance, men—even today—rely more consistently on bows and arrows. In contrast, women are much more likely to have a variety of preferences: Some of them are partial to knives, some use bows and arrows, and others use a combination. And while men typically hunted as a solitary pursuit or with a single partner, women hunted cooperatively, even socially—with other women, children, and groups of dogs.

In our present times, the myth of the exclusively male hunter hasn't gone away. Meat is still considered masculine. We talk about manning the barbecue grill—and more often or not, it *is* a man flipping the burgers and searing the steaks—while ConAgra Foods' ground-beef sandwich mix is still marketed as Manwich. (I can remember cringing when a lawyer described the compensation system at his firm in which each partner brings home the share of the revenues they created as the "eat what we kill" model.)

This idea that meat is manly has no doubt been promulgated by a society that benefits a masculine sense of superiority, where the man needs protein to be strong and hustles to find it while a woman orders the salad.

Meanwhile, prehistoric women weren't just wielding spears and going in for the kill; they had parity with men in other ways, demonstrating strategic leadership roles early on.

To give an example: When over a century ago archaeologists first began excavating a tenth-century grave in Birka, Sweden, they believed that they had discovered the remains of a high-ranking official.[5] The grave, known as Bj 581, contained not only a body but also weapons, shields, horses, and a kind of strategic board game, which pointed to the site being the final resting place of someone involved in wartime tactics, a great warrior who led troops. When the grave was discovered a hundred years ago, people thought warriors of such rank were men, so the skeleton was assumed to belong to a man. It wasn't until 2017, after researchers took DNA from teeth and arm bones from the grave, that they learned that this particular warrior had X chromosomes, without any sign of a Y. An analysis of the isotopes gave further clues, including that this female Viking badass was probably over thirty when she died and well-traveled, that she was likely a respected leader.[6]

I don't blame the archaeologists. I would have assumed the Viking was a man, too. Because in this world, we carry countless assumptions when it comes to how we view gender. I'm reminded of this when I wear a sleeveless dress and my arms elicit comments of surprise or discomfort. "Oh my god, you are jacked," a colleague said to me once, with a hint of gloom, warning, displeasure, or discomfort in the voice—maybe a mix of all of these. My burly muscles subvert a gender norm. Much like the Viking warrior, lying quietly in the grave waiting for someone to notice that "he" was in fact "she."

Data Reveals Women Crushing It

Women's bodies are extraordinary and work in ways we're only beginning to understand. Have you ever had that feeling—during a race or some other competition—of just hitting your stride while the others were starting to peter out? That's how women's bodies work compared to men's. Sure, a man might be able to lift a bigger rock than a woman, but when researchers in Scotland and Canada compared weightlifting exercises at percentages of maximal strength among a group of men and women, they found that, in several instances, women could outlast men when it came to exercises performed at an equal percent of their max— making a strong case for female endurance capabilities.[7] The ability of women to outlast men was most apparent in exercises performed at low intensities of around 20 percent of maximal strength, says researcher Ron Maughan, now a visiting professor at the University of St. Andrews.

In the 1980s, Maughan studied and compared raw strength in men versus women. And while most men were stronger than women, there were also plenty of women who were stronger than men—and worthy of further study. "Everyone says men are stronger than women, and it's complete nonsense," says Maughan. "There's an awful lot of women who are stronger than most men."

The problem is that most scientific research has historically focused on men. We are only just learning about the true extent of women's strengths, which have long been overlooked in a society powered by men exerting their dominance. One 2021 paper looked at all the sports science research covered in six journals between 2014 and 2020 and found that of the more than five thousand studies with 12.5 million participants, only one-third were female.[8]

To give another example: In the past, it was assumed that men had faster oxygen uptake than women. Then, in 2017, Thomas Beltrame from the University of Waterloo in Canada led the research that compared women's oxygen uptake during aerobic activity with men's. (In previous studies, the sample pool mixed both men and women.) Beltrame and colleagues Richard L. Hughson and Rodrigo Villar recruited eighteen healthy young participants: nine male and nine female. All participants were highly active, paired by similar ages and BMI, and were asked to engage in several treadmill exercise tests of various intensities. The tests revealed that oxygen extraction dynamics were remarkably faster in women than men, which led to better aerobic fitness, Beltrame says.[9]

These advantages can and should be explored further to be understood, expanded upon, and maximized. For all we know, we might have only scratched the surface of what women are capable of, and with some better research and understanding, we could train ourselves to do much more. Maybe these inherent female advantages can be pushed much, much further.

One of the reasons that data on female performance is sorely lacking is that men have participated in sports in more significant numbers over a more extended period, which has skewed the data and representative sample sizes. For instance, women could not officially compete in marathons until the 1970s. In 1967, twenty-year-old Kathrine Switzer, a student at Syracuse University, registered for the Boston Marathon under the name K. V. Switzer. While there were no official rules against women entering the race, it also was something that wasn't done—and it didn't even occur to anyone watching that Switzer was a female until the second mile of the race. When officials discovered Switzer was a woman, the race manager Jock Semple attempted to push her off the course.

"So much of research in science and medicine is really based on men and male cohorts, especially in sports performance," explained Clara Wu Tsai in a November 2023 interview with *The Washington Post*.[10] Together with her husband, Alibaba cofounder Joe Tsai, Wu Tsai owns two professional basketball teams, including the New York Liberty Women's National Basketball Association team. With a keen interest in women athletes, she has funded a program to encourage more studies on what makes female athletes tick—including energy levels, the effects of hormones, menses, menopause, resilience, and energy. Female athletes, she points out, have never really been studied as a cohort. Meanwhile, they are likelier to suffer ACL injuries at two to eight times the rate of men,[11] experience higher rates of concussion,[12] and are more likely to suffer long-term negative consequences of those injuries, such as early-onset osteoarthritis.[13] Further, one in three girls drops out of sports by her late teens, compared to just one in ten teenage boys.[14] The Female Athlete Program studies why and tries to develop therapies and preventive techniques.

Meanwhile, scientists at the Salk Institute, a recipient of the Tsais' funding, are mapping the molecules and gene expression changes in athletes during performance, healing, and recovery. The goal: To create an "interactive blueprint"—at the molecular and cellular level—that determines how human performance differs in men versus women. The findings have already shown dozens of sex-related differences, which will provide fresh insight into how men and women adapt to training, rejuvenate while sleeping, adjust with age, respond to nutrients, and repair upon injury.[15]

For instance, muscle biopsies demonstrate a higher density of capillaries in women.[16] Certain types of muscle are more resistant to fatigue, and women have more of those than men.[17] And though females typically have smaller lungs and airways, their diaphragms are more fatigue-resistant.[18] Researchers argue that this can affect how and what types of exercise can and should be prescribed therapeutically to women as opposed to men. It may also lead to more appropriate, better-targeted systems of training.

Female athletes are unique from men in that their hormones fluctuate in a constant monthly cycle related to reproduction, and levels of estrogen and progesterone can quickly get out of whack with too much exercise, stress, and poor diet. It gets worse, as girls are in a time of their lives when they are faced with excessive body pressures over how they look. What's known as the female athlete triad is a combination of three conditions: menstrual dysfunction, low energy availability (with or without an eating disorder), and decreased bone mineral density. It is relatively common among young women participating in sports. The American College of Sports Medicine first identified it in 1992, and the intertwined clinical conditions are still in their nascency of being understood.[19] In more recent years, the more comprehensive term *relative energy deficiency in sport*, or RED-S, has become used to describe a broader set of symptoms beyond menstrual and bone health. Diagnosing and treating the issues can be complicated and may involve more than one specialist.

Kathryn E. Ackerman, medical director of the Female Athlete Program in the Orthopedics and Sports Medicine Department at Boston Children's Hospital, says myriad considerations make this combination of symptoms challenging to study and understand. Coaches don't typically want to address periods with their athletes. It's also important to be careful about talking about weight with that population—for instance, when using terms like *making weight* for a lightweight team.

Olympic figure skater Rachael Flatt says she received many messages about her weight while growing up in a sport that emphasizes thinness. When she ascended onto the national stage at age twelve, her body began filling out as she entered puberty.

"The women at the top had very lean and svelte body types," recalls Flatt. "As my body started changing, I remember thinking I needed to make sure my body looked the way theirs did," she says.

She was reprimanded for not meeting a body standard—by coaches, judges, and the general public. Costume fittings emphasized "extending your line," she recalls—code for making her legs appear thinner. Her coach once told her that she would have an easier time completing a routine if she weren't "carrying a sack of potatoes," she says. Judges even suggested she lose twenty pounds mere weeks before a world championship. And commentary on social media accused her of putting on the "freshman fifteen."

The punishing self-talk in her head was strong because the messages around her were relentless. While she believes she never developed a full-threshold eating disorder, she found herself restricting food and exercising extensively if she felt she overate. "A lot of those comments will stick with me forever," says Flatt, now a thirty-two-year-old clinical psychologist with a special interest in studying disordered eating and helping athletes with body image problems.

"Without those experiences," she says, "I wouldn't be doing what I am doing today."

Looking ahead is so important for young women. We lose a lot of our bone mass once we hit menopause, so it's incumbent on medical providers, coaches, and nutritionists to communicate the value of calcium, magnesium, vitamin D, and good nutrition. "If you wait to fix the nutritional issue until you're thirty, you can't make up those losses from your teens and twenties," says Dr. Ackerman in Boston. Knowledge is power, and if we don't have enough information or lack knowledgeable people around to advise us, we will continue to be at a severe disadvantage.

Adam Is Different from Eve

Of course, widely accepted differences between men and women put them into one of two categories. But the reality is more shaded, driven by biology and society. Gender falls within a spectrum. Typically, men have more muscle mass, bigger hearts, and more lung capacity. But plenty of women also cross into that male range and vice versa. Estrogen has a protective effect on muscle fibers and cell membranes, and it also improves fat metabolism. During exercise, estrogen primes the body to use stored fat before carbohydrates. Fat, which contains more calories than carbs, burns more slowly, which delays fatigue during endurance activities. Female bodies tend to be better equipped for extreme endurance activities[20]—perhaps one way Mother Nature has adapted women to the ever-exhausting roles of mother, caretaker, nurse, and best friend among countless tribes across generations.

Testosterone gets all the attention when it comes to athleticism. It's the male hormone associated with advantages in the sports and fitness world, but women have testosterone, too. And on the flip side, estrogen—which females make more of than males do—actually plays a critical role in athletic performance, but in a more subtle way. While testosterone amplifies speed and strength, estrogen influences fine motor skills and coordination. While men excel at short bursts of power, women are better suited for endurance—and estrogen is part of the reason.

In addition, the types of muscle fibers differ between women and men. While men have more fast-twitch (or type II) fibers, those associated with short, powerful bursts of strength, women have more slow-twitch (type I) fibers. These latter types of fibers, which are likelier to use fat for a slow burn of energy, are not as quick-hit powerful, but take a longer time to tire—making them great for staying the course. Men's fast-twitch fibers, on the other hand, take up carbohydrates for quick energy and power, but also tire more quickly.

Men have bigger hearts and greater lung capacity and more upper-body strength. Still, even so, research shows that women are more resistant to fatigue than men, which means they can perform at the same relative intensity for a longer duration. In a 2016 review of more than fifty-five fatigue studies published between 1972 and 2015, women were shown, on average, to outlast men by 36 percent in exercises that measured stamina (i.e., how long they could hold a contraction with arm or leg muscles).[21]

"In terms of sheer strength, yes, males are stronger than females. But ask them to sustain that strength over a period of time, and females will typically outperform men," explains study author Sandra Hunter, chair of movement science in the School of Kinesiology at the University of Michigan–Ann Arbor. Some of her studies show that women retain more strength in their legs after running or cycling for an extended period. She points to sex differences in the makeup of the muscle tissue: "Males tend to have larger, but more fatigable fibers," she says.

And let's not forget the statistics showing the extent to which women live longer than men. These are remarkable and indisputable: The global life expectancy at birth for a woman is seventy-six, compared with seventy-one for a man.[22] More than three-fourths of centenarians are women.[23] At older ages, the ratio is even higher: As of October 4, 2024, there were 310 validated supercentenarians (people who are at least 110 years old) in the world, according to the Gerontology Research Group. The first sixty-two people on the list are all women; they range in age from 112 to 116. Then John Tinniswood of England shows up at number sixty-three.[24]

Women's superior life expectancy is "one of the most robust features of human biology that we know," says Steven Austad, former chair of the biology department at the University of Alabama at Birmingham and scientific director of the American Federation for Aging Research. For the past twenty years, Austad has tried to unravel the mystery of why women live longer than men. His work analyzes human mortality data from as far back as records have been kept and from all over the world. And his findings show that women outlive men by anywhere from 5 percent to 20 percent.[25]

The self-described data nerd has plumbed the Human Mortality Database, which provides detailed historical population records from more than thirty countries. He says that in every one of those countries, women showed greater life expectancy at birth than men and for every year on record. He uses Sweden as an example, as this is a country with more complete and reliable records than anyplace else on earth: Beginning back in 1800, when life expectancy at birth was thirty-three years for women and thirty-one years for men, Swedish women have lived longer than men every single year all the way to today, when they live to eighty-five years on average, while men only live to an average of eighty-two.

The data illustrate a story of survivorship: There are 105 males born per 100 females. By around age fifteen, the numbers even out, with more males dying early deaths. After that, populations skew slightly more female. That pattern is seen in every country in every year for which reliable birth and death records exist, Austad says. "There may be no more robust pattern in human biology," he writes.[26]

This also plays out in how men and women are affected by disease. In the United States, women have historically died at lower rates than men in fourteen of the top fifteen causes of death, according to Austad's review of the Human Mortality Database. Women died at higher rates than men only of Alzheimer's disease.[27]

All of which raises the question: Is there something inherent in women's genetic makeup that is advantageous? One theory is that because women have two X chromosomes, this gives them an edge, with a copy if one gene is defective. Neonatologists even say that premature male babies have lower survival rates than female babies. "Even prenatally, there seems to be more toughness in females than in males," Austad says.

Other hypotheses: Austad says there are some indications that women have a more responsive immune system than men.

Another possibility is that sex hormones may be involved. Either men's reproductive hormones increase their susceptibility to disease or women's hormones provide them with greater resistance. Some evidence even points to the possibility of the life-shortening impact of men's hormones. Longevity records from eighty-one Korean eunuchs who resided at the royal court in the sixteenth to the nineteenth centuries show that eunuchs lived fifteen to twenty years longer than modern (intact) men. Similarly, records recovered from a mental institution in the 1940s where castrations were performed for behavioral reasons showed that on average the nearly 300 castrated men lived 13.6 years longer than the 735 intact men.

"There is so much available data," Austad says. "The more you dig into the data, the more and more female advantages you come across."

Austad doesn't deal just with human data; he also looks at animal data. His investigation into monkeys and apes revealed some interesting insights. Female apes and monkeys are generally longer-lived than males in wild populations. But in captive populations, particularly those where males contribute significantly to parental care, captive males can live longer than captive females.

One hypothesis, Austad says, is that caretaking helps build a robustness—and the associated longevity might be a benefit to the lead role that women take in caring for others.

When it comes to us humans, scientists are only beginning to understand male versus female forms of aggression. Most existing research into the fight-or-flight response—in which the sympathetic nervous system activates a hormonal cascade of norepinephrine and epinephrine—involves calculating whether an animal has a realistic chance of overcoming a predator. For a guy, that's a pretty straightforward calculation: Yapping dog on a leash? I'm probably okay. Big tiger? Let's get out of here.

Before 1995, women constituted only about 17 percent of participants in laboratory studies of physiological and neuroendocrine responses to stress. Researchers who study fight-or-flight responses in males and females have theorized that childbearing and being the primary caregiver for successive generations may have adapted the instinct differently in women. Rather than throwing up our fists or choosing to run, we seem to be hardwired to think protectively, because we can carry and produce offspring, then nurse and tend to them. Women have spent a lot of time fine-tuning the behaviors that increase our babies' survival: shushing them, calming them, getting them out of the way, or retrieving them from something that could hurt them. We don't just throw ourselves into a fight or flee.

So how has this evolved the way women do aggression? In some ways, the answer to this question reveals the ways we are in fact even stronger and smarter than men: We play the long game and think strategically. Males are more likely to use physical aggression during power struggles or to show off in front of their friends. But females take a more cerebral approach, using social networks to enlist others and form alliances. For generations, women have been affiliating themselves with social groups to reduce risk. The process of befriending, researchers say, is made up of networks created by females and for females and their offspring. It follows that neuroendocrine mechanisms would have evolved to regulate these responses to stress, much as sympathetic activation is thought to provide the physiological basis for the fight-or-flight response. All these underpinnings of the attachment/caregiving system, the thinking goes, may feed into the way we respond to stress and the way we view our own strength.[28]

All of which is to say, our bodies are extraordinary, operating on a much higher level than those of our male counterparts, leading us to work collaboratively and strategically instead of simply putting up our dukes. We can deliver life into the world. We live longer than men. And we have more endurance than men. If you think about it for long enough, it's utterly crazy that women have been pigeonholed for so long as inferior, weaker, and second class and that, at least here in the United States, we have waited so long to see a female leader of this country while we earn 82 percent of what men do. (Black women, by the way, earn only 70 percent as much as white men, and Hispanic women earn only 65 percent.) We still have to fight for representation on corporate boards and in sports, even if studies consistently show that we're tougher, can last longer, and can and will crush the competition, given half the chance.

CHAPTER 3

LIFT HEAVY THINGS

The Science of Strong, from the Great Sandwina to
the Gorgeous Ladies of Wrestling

My coach, a pint-size retired professional bodybuilder named
Tina Peratino, altered the way I think about exercise. Tina, a
four-foot-eleven-and-a-half ex-physique competitor who coaches
from her Bowie, Maryland, home, set me on a path of intense
daily workouts and a new approach to how I ate, how I stocked
my fridge, and how I fed both myself and my family. Within
two months, I was hooked. For so long, I had carried around a
list of assumptions in my head—stuff I had read in fitness magazines or on food packaging. These included: cardio good, weights
bad; eat less; order the salad, eliminate carbs; bananas make you
fat. I had similar preconceived notions about lifting. Could hoisting weights create a torso that would look bad in a sundress?

Would my voice start to get lower? Tina explained to me that I needed to unlearn what I thought I knew, assumed, or imagined.

Working with Tina upended a belief I had held for a very long time: that to be thin meant success. That thinness was power. That it signified I was finally good enough. Getting involved in weightlifting helped me to understand how incredibly false that pervasive conceit was.

From our first meeting in the mirrored posing room she uses for her training sessions, I saw something valuable in Tina's example. She was beautiful, but not by that long-held standard of physical fragility. In fact, the first thing I noticed was not her thinness or lack of it. That didn't register. Tina looked strong, powerful, and confident. She was a butterfly freed from some kind of cage. The sight of her flipped a switch in my mind, and as a result, my ideal body image shifted.

As I learned more about the world of bodybuilding, I discovered that there was a lot of science to back up the power and confidence Tina exuded—and how I was beginning to feel myself. Muscle is the secret sauce to a longer and stronger existence. Building more of it is what keeps our physical frame not only looking young but acting it as well. It is the infrastructure that holds the key to all kinds of activities—from climbing stairs to playing with children, hiking with a partner, maneuvering around accidents, being able to lift household objects, and preventing falls—that ultimately lead to a better life. A major reason muscle is so critical for women is the necessity of muscle mass for our bones. Muscle is a bone's best friend, acting as a cushion and a protector.

Strength is something we take for granted when we are young, and it increases up to around the age of thirty.[1] After that, muscle power and performance begin a slow and steady decline, decreasing with age at the rate of about 3 to 8 percent per decade[2]—a slide that accelerates after menopause with the loss of estrogen. After age fifty, bone breakdown outpaces bone formation, and bone loss accelerates.[3] Studies have shown that strength training not only helps slow bone loss but can also build bone.[4] Activities that put stress on bones cause cells to form more bone matter. That stress comes from the impact on bones that can occur during strength training and other weight-bearing exercises like running. The result amounts to bones that are both stronger and denser.[5]

Building muscle also increases metabolism. As women age, their metabolism slows down, which can lead to a steady weight gain. The pounds pile on at about the rate of one and a half pounds each year as a woman goes through her fifties.[6] Hormonal changes are in part the culprit, as fat tends to develop around the midsection rather than hips and thighs.

Conversely, a muscular physique reshapes how the body works, making it function better and more efficiently: While muscle doesn't directly burn fat, the more muscle mass you have, the higher your basal metabolic rate (the number of calories the body needs to perform basic functions that keep you alive, like breathing). This means that—without any further exercising—women with more muscle typically burn more calories throughout the day. A higher metabolic rate burns more calories constantly, even at rest.[7]

And research also validates the sense of empowerment and achievement that I experienced when building muscle. Resistance training, as with other types of exercise such as running and swimming, can significantly increase a type of protein called brain-derived neurotrophic factor (BDNF) in the hippocampus area of the brain. The hippocampus is responsible for mood, memory, and other cognitive functions, and in people who are struggling with feelings of depression, it actually gets smaller. The release of BDNF spurs new brain cells in the hippocampus, helping to grow it back.[8]

The practice of exercise increases blood flow and oxygen to the brain, as well as the release of endorphins and serotonin, which are neurotransmitters that contribute to feelings of happiness. They are otherwise known as "feel good" hormones. When you feel good inside and out, you naturally project yourself more confidently in the world.

Historically, studies exploring the relationship between exercise and mental health have focused on aerobic activity. There may be several reasons for this. For one thing, it is easier to study aerobic activity than the movement of muscle you can't even see. Results such as maximal oxygen uptake scores are more easily obtained when those being tested are on machines like digital treadmills and ellipticals; inputs can be fine-tuned, observation windows are usually longer, and data can be more immediately extracted. Accurately assessing strength gains can be more complicated. At the same time, aerobic exercise is most people's workout of choice—not only is it relatively easy to lace up your sneakers and get moving, but cardio is an effective way to burn fat, a primary concern for many people. But a 2018 study published in *JAMA Psychiatry* analyzed thirty-three clinical trials for the effects of resistance exercise (more specifically, weightlifting) on depression. Results showed that these strength building workouts significantly reduced depressive symptoms among research participants—similar to long-standing results reported with aerobic exercise.[9]

Studies have found that weightlifting benefits the brain in other ways, too. For instance Georgia Tech researchers found that a single bout of lifting weights can improve memory.[10] Researchers investigated whether a series of single-leg knee extensions could produce memory benefits forty-eight hours later among a group of twenty-three adults compared with a group of twenty-three adults who did not exercise. After both groups were tested with a series of image-recollection exercises, researchers found that the active group had about 20 percent higher overall recognition accuracy than the group that did not exercise.

This chimes with my personal experience. Before I found weightlifting, I was at the mercy of my moods, experiencing waves of depression and feelings of powerlessness. Now that weights are a part of my life, I rely on the mood boost I get from working out. These days, I always exercise around eleven a.m. or three p.m.—after the morning crush or before the five p.m. gym rush hour. Whether I exercise in my basement or a commercial gym, I enter feeling fine. But afterward, I feel like a much-improved version of myself. I come back to my desk smarter, stronger, and more centered.

A muscular physique reshapes how the body works, making it function better and more efficiently. "When you are strength training, you are structuring a bigger engine for burning fat," explains Edward Laskowski, a specialist in sports medicine at the Mayo Clinic, in an interview with me.[11] The reason so many diets plateau, he says, is because we tend to focus solely on food and cardio at the expense of weights. It doesn't need to take a ton of time to achieve the positive effect of lifting weights, he adds. The key is pushing the muscle to fatigue. That can be done in ten to twenty minutes. The important thing is to do it regularly. And not every workout has to be a drop-dead, all-or-nothing, "fall to exhaustion in a sweat puddle" type of affair. (Mine rarely are. Most often they feel like I got a good lift in, then I'm done.) Most coaches will tell you that consistency, rather than any particular workout, matters the most.

For me, the number one thing that helped me with consistency was finding a community of women who were also committed to making weights a part of their daily lives. I enjoy being part of a team Facebook group, where recipes, training progress, weight-room stories, and competition results are shared. While we are all from different walks of life, political leanings, and opinions, we share the same coach and feel like we are part of a team. We have developed a real camaraderie. The reality is that women have always formed subcultures of empowerment that buck a traditional male-dominated view of what's attractive or desirable in this way—we just don't always get to hear about them. In fact, there's an entire alternative history waiting to be told that doesn't focus on women's fragility or delicacy, but on their tremendous strength and power instead.

The Great Sandwina

The precursors to modern-day bodybuilders were so-called strongwomen in the nineteenth century, who tended to appear in sideshows and circuses, where they would show off their superhuman prowess as entertainment. In other words, women who sought to buck convention by lifting weights.

Take Katie Brumbach, who was also known as the Great Sandwina. She was born in 1884 in Essen, Germany, to parents who were Viennese circus performers and who incorporated their children into their husband-and-wife strongman and strongwoman act. At the turn of the century, Katie married acrobat Max Heymann. She capably incorporated her new husband into an act involving lifting him over her head with one arm—sometimes with weights or with her son. She began billing herself as the Great Sandwina (an apparent jab at Eugen Sandow, the German bodybuilding pioneer billed as the "Perfect Man," whom she defeated in a contest in 1902 when she lifted three hundred pounds over her head, which Sandow could only get to his chest).

Katie and Max soon took their act to America, where she was billed as Europe's Queen of Strength and Beauty, Lady Hercules, and the Strongest Woman in the World. Later, she joined the Ringling Bros. and Barnum & Bailey Circus as a powerlifter, where she snapped iron bars with her bare hands. She was succeeded by others who turned their athleticism into performance art, including Ivy Russell and Luisita Leers.

Charlotte Perkins Gilman

For other women at the turn of the century, building one's body became a refuge during a time when many women felt trapped by patriarchal conventions. In some cases, these women quietly discovered sports, organized themselves into teams, and built gyms in defiance of a society that wanted them to be quiet and hold still. The novelist and feminist Charlotte Perkins Gilman, born in 1860, was one of these women. As well as being an accomplished author of classic texts such as the short story "The Yellow Wallpaper," she was instrumental in founding the Sanitary Gymnasium for Ladies and Children in Providence, Rhode Island, a women's gym modeled after a similar one in Boston. The gym became a huge hit, attracting women from throughout the area who, in the words of Gilman, wanted to "wear abbreviated garments and elevate the massive dumbbell at our leisure." The gym was advertised as a place where women could "Broaden Narrow Chests and Strengthen Weak Muscles" and provide the "Movement Cure for the Treatment of Extreme Nervous Prostration When All Other Means Fail." For Gilman and the other women who worked out at the gymnasium, athleticism was a way to improve not only the body but also the mind and the nervous system.

This was a time when many women suffered with what we would call stress, anxiety, and depression, but which back then was known by the blanket term *neurasthenia*. Medical doctors at the time often blamed neurasthenia on recent social changes: the burgeoning women's suffrage movement, as well as young women entering higher education and careers in greater numbers and doing the kind of cerebral work that kept them out of the home. The remedy most often prescribed for cases of neurasthenia was rest. Doctors were literally telling women not to leave the house, to go back to bed and stay there.

From an early age, Gilman had struggled with depression,

but had found that exercise and weightlifting helped alleviate her symptoms. She had become a devotee of the work of William Blaikie, a New York lawyer and athlete who had written the 1879 book *How to Get Strong and How to Stay So.* In her diary, she wrote: "Follow Blaikie every night with the greatest assiduity. I can put all my fingers on the floor, knees straight to count of 30." As a student at the Rhode Island School of Design, she became a self-taught athlete, forging her own training, skipping taking the easy way to class and "running up the whole four flights two steps at a time, beating the elevator, to my immense satisfaction."[12]

Enamored with athleticism and its effects on her mental health, she convinced a local gym operator, Dr. J. P. Brooks, to open a ladies-only gym. Brooks wasn't convinced enough women would want to join, but Gilman was insistent. When she asked him how many he'd need, he said, "About thirty," so she rounded them up. The Sanitary Gymnasium was born, its goal to "promote a healthful use of gymnastic exercise among ladies and children." Gilman worked out at the gym multiple times a week, sometimes daily, often adding dumbbells to her workout. Her favorite activity was swinging on suspended rings, which she described as "near to flying as one gets, outside of a circus." She came up with new garments for her workouts—long chemises, pantaloons, and an early version of a brassiere—that made athletic movement easier.

Sadly, Gilman's daily workouts soon came to a halt. She got married in 1884 and stopped going to the gym, deciding that exercise and strong ambitions were not appropriate for a housewife and soon-to-be mother. So she gave up athletics, and after the birth of her first child, suffered from a debilitating depression, which we would probably call postpartum depression today. Under her doctor's orders, she stayed in her bed, which only made her feel worse. Eventually, she published her now-acclaimed short story "The Yellow Wallpaper" in 1892, which describes a woman's descent into madness while on a "rest cure."

Pudgy Stockton

It wasn't until the early twentieth century that we had a real vision of women's strength in the form of Abbye "Pudgy" Stockton, the first true female bodybuilder. Stockton was born Abbye Eville in 1917 and spent most of her life in Southern California. She was nicknamed Pudgy as a child, a moniker that stuck. After graduating from high school, she got a job answering telephones in Los Angeles, but as soon as she was finished for the day, she made straight for the beach. In the late 1930s, there was an outdoor venue in Santa Monica just south of the pier, where acrobats and a variety of stunt performers practiced their acts for films, and where Pudgy liked to hang out. It became an attraction for beachgoers and athletes who liked to watch and participate. (Later, in the 1940s, the area became known as Muscle Beach.) In 1941, Pudgy married Les Stockton, who was an athlete and performer in the Muscle Beach community. They formed hand-balancing acts with friends. Pudgy held her husband above her head in a handstand and she balanced off her husband's extended arms holding a one-hundred-pound dumbbell.[13]

She became known as the Queen of Muscle Beach and in 1944 started writing a column for a fitness magazine called *Strength and Health*, which she continued turning out every month until

1954. The column, called "Barbelles," was written for women interested in training for muscle. "In those days, lifting weights was considered unfeminine," Stockton later explained in an interview with *Sports Illustrated Women*. "People used to say that if women worked out, they would become masculine looking or wouldn't be able to get pregnant. We just laughed because we knew they were wrong."[14] In 1947, she also organized the first Amateur Athletic Union–sanctioned weightlifting meet for women, taking the notion of female bodybuilding out of the realm of circus act to the level of a respected sport. In doing so, she also showed that weightlifting to build a strong muscular physique was sexy and aesthetically appealing.

Stockton appeared on over forty magazine covers and also posed with the best male bodybuilders of the era, such as John Grimek and Steve Reeves. Muscle Beach grew, in no small part thanks to Pudgy and her performances and columns. The city of Santa Monica put up various gymnastic tools, including rings, bars, and platforms at the beach. Les went to serve in World War II, and when he returned home, the couple opened up their own health clubs, including one for women only called the Salon of Figure Development.[15]

Pudgy was also one of the first women to wear a two-piece bathing suit, to allow easier movement in gymnastic stunts. "You couldn't buy a two-piece, so my mother ripped apart an old brassiere to use as a pattern," recalled Stockton in a 1988 interview with the *Los Angeles Times*.[16] She was soon having the two-piece suits custom-made for her.

Pudgy's iconic status catapulted interest in a feminine form that reflected the possibilities of what women could accomplish athletically. But it wasn't until 1972, with the signing of Title IX of the Education Amendments, which provided for equal treatment of the sexes in educational settings, that we could really see the growth of women in U.S. sports. And from there, popular interest grew in a female physique that showed the signs of a hard-earned athleticism, with the first-ever competition for women bodybuilders taking place in Canton, Ohio, in 1977.

Derby Girls

As is often the case, women tend to be at the forefront of new sports, pushing boundaries even as they're continually told not to. Besides the world of bodybuilding, another community of kick-ass women bucking the standard notions of body ideal can be found in competitive roller derby, a contact sport where full, muscular figures are championed and celebrated. Unabashedly thrusting their hips and butts to outlast their opponents, wearing fishnet stockings and tattoos, the brazen athletes in this arena mix unabashed sex appeal with colorful nicknames like Miss Fortune, Road Rage, and One-Hit Wonder.

Roller Derby was initially a product of the 1930s, when audiences during the Depression were looking for new and thrilling forms of entertainment. Event promoter Leo Seltzer and journalist Damon Runyon are credited with taking the roller-skating marathons that were popular at the time and creating the full-contact entertainment sport of roller derby as it's known today. In a bout, or match, ten skaters take to the track with five players on each team. The team consists of a jammer, whose job is to overtake laps on the other team to earn points, and four blockers, who try to stop the other team's jammer. Each round—or jam—begins with a race between the two jammers and goes for two minutes. Teams get points when their jammer laps an opponent.[17]

By 1949, roller derby had become a national sensation, with both men and women skating. ABC broadcast the bouts up to three times a week. Mickey Rooney starred in the 1950 film *The Fireball* (which also featured a young Marilyn Monroe) about a runaway orphan turned roller-derby champion.[18]

But it was the women who stole the show. Gerry Murray and Midge "Toughie" Brasuhn became household names, their personalities and prowess exhilarating to fans, and their rivalry legendary. In 1950, Brasuhn was voted one of the country's ten outstanding women in sports by sportswriters.

Murray, who played for most of her career with the New York Chiefs, was "a female terror, swishing around the track at 30 miles an hour, hipping her opponents, zigzagging recklessly, her red hair, tied in a ribbon, winging along behind her," Gay Talese wrote in *The New York Times* in 1958.[19]

"The worst roughing up I got was in Chicago against Toughie," Murray told the gossip columnist Earl Wilson in 1950 about the serious leg injury she incurred in one of their bruising encounters. "She gave me one of those terrific blocks and I wasn't even expecting it. I ended up on the rail. I hit the upright in midair."[20] (Off the track, the two women were known to be good friends.)

Jessica Strübel, a consumer psychology professor at the University of Rhode Island who researches women and body image, cowrote a paper called "'Bout Time! Renegotiating the Body in Roller Derby."[21] Strübel says she was initially struck by a group of derby women she noticed piling into a Dallas dive bar after a match one summer day in 2014. They were wearing fishnets and tight crop tops with their names and numbers on the back. "They were loud and brash and having fun. I was just taken by how cool they looked, and being somebody who studies body image, I was struck by how they were larger, super confident and wearing skimpy clothes–and owning it . . . I was surprised, in a good way, and drawn in about everything that this environment provided to women."[22] In doing research for the paper, she surveyed sixty-four roller-derby women. On average, they responded more positively to questions about their weight and physical condition than nonparticipants in the sport.

Roller derby, argued Strubel, encourages women to be comfortable with their bodies and sexual assertiveness "in a society that advocates a hetero-femininity through the media and even in traditional sports where women are often marginalized and still expected to be physically weaker and inferior to men."

I tested this myself by interviewing roller-derby participants, to see what attracted them to the sport and the impact that it had. One of the women I spoke with, Sara LeMay, a thirty-year old accountant in Colorado Springs, Colorado, says the sport has really helped her find positive attributes about her body, something that she had struggled with since her teenage years.

"In high school I was always bottom heavy," says LeMay. "I was self-conscious about it. I was a size eight. They called me the girl with the butt."

As a teen, she had been an inline speed skater and roller hockey player. One summer, she started playing roller derby at Skateland, a roller rink in Olympia, Washington, where she went to practice and to work at the snack bar. In 2010 when she turned eighteen, she joined the Oly Rollers team, made up of three to four dozen women ranging from their late teens to mid-forties who trained six hours a week. "We were competitive and hard-hitting," LeMay explains.

The Oly Rollers came in all shapes and sizes. They were jovial and proud of their wry, badass aesthetic. They adopted special nicknames highlighting a dark or tough side to their personalities; some wore fishnets and skirts or torn-jean shorts to games. And while LeMay says she favors more traditional athletic gear to play in—leggings or yoga pants and a jersey—she has embraced a roller-derby name: Scara to Death. When she was growing up, the boys on her hockey team called her Scara—as an insult—which she loathed. "Now I embraced this nickname that I'd hated my entire life," she says. "It was an opportunity to own it."

More than this, though, the sport—and being around the women in it—"has helped define for me what a healthy body is," she says. Rather than seeing her physique as an anomaly, she now views it as an asset. In her position as a pivot, she is charged with blocking the opposition from the other team. "Having more weight behind my hips is better than being super tiny," she says.

Fight Club: The Gorgeous Ladies of Wrestling

In my search to find alternative body ideals to the standard skinny, I inevitably came upon the women of the Gorgeous Ladies of Wrestling, or GLOW. Founded in 1985 by wrestling promoter David McLane, GLOW was the first full-time American women's wrestling company to have a regular television program. This aired weekly as an entertainment show featuring character-driven stories and rowdy sketches performed on the wrestling mat. Besides feuds in the ring, the individual characters sang rap songs and participated in comedy skits.

The women involved in GLOW were primarily actresses, models, dancers, and stunt performers trying to break into show business. The pilot episode for the TV show was taped on December 5, 1985, in Las Vegas and the program debuted in syndication on September 13, 1986.[23] Regular characters included Hollywood, Vine, Col. Ninotchka, Sally, the Farmer's Daughter, and Mountain Fiji. For children of the 1980s, it was the first time that we saw women throwing each other around, hurling hits, looking angry and unladylike.

Jackie Stallone, mother of Sylvester, appeared on the show periodically as the manager of Stallone's Sweethearts (the "good girl" faction of wrestlers), while Kitty Burke managed the "bad girls."

In late 1987, David McLane, who had wanted to focus his GLOW product more on in-ring action, left the show in a dispute with its producers. He went back to Indianapolis along with some of the original GLOW girls. In 1988 a new season debuted with a next generation of stars competing alongside the remaining GLOW originals. Production eventually ended after four seasons and 104 episodes in 1990.[24]

Nearly thirty years later, a fictionalized version of the show called GLOW resurfaced as a series on Netflix, helmed by writers Liz Flahive and Carly Mensch, which followed the lives of the stars inside and outside the ring. Mensch says she was taken by the incongruity of a male-centric concept. The plan was to sex-ualize and make women appear cartoonish by putting them in a wrestling ring for the public to gawk at, but that as this was done, the women took ownership of their roles and found strength in them, really driving the show.

"It was exploitation and empowerment at the same time," said showrunner Carly Mensch in an interview with me. "We were taken by the contradiction—that men hired these women based on who they thought was pretty or strong or could be the right type or whatever," she says. "But the women took it from there."[25]

The Dissonance-Based Intervention

Women like the wrestlers of *GLOW* have always found ways to upend the traditional male-dominated view of what's attractive or desirable. It's along these edges of what's commercially beau-tiful or acceptable that certain communities of women have banded together to chip away at the false idol of skinny. These women take up space, literally and figuratively; they claim their power. They've created countercultures of confidence, from booty songs in hip-hop culture to body positivity proponents on social media. In one viral video, content creator and self-described body-acceptance advocate Marissa Matthews responds to a comment that "everyone has time to lose weight," by saying, "I can't understand why I can't just exist in my body." TikTok has been a way for people to share ideas and feelings about bodies and bigness. In another video, Lizzo says, "Our bodies are none of your fucking business. Our health is none of your fucking business."

I spoke with a CrossFit competitor from Niceville, Florida, about how her body confidence has changed over the years. Quinn Padilla is proud of her thighs, her favorite thing about her body nowadays. They're big. They're muscular. They're badass. For a long time, her Instagram handle was @QuadsLikeQuinn. But it wasn't always the case: The thirty-six-year-old therapist and mother of three recalls hating her legs so much that she would sit a certain way at school to make her legs look thinner.

"I'd sit on my tiptoes," she says. "I hated the way my big thighs would smash onto the seat."

Quinn grew up seeing the women in her family struggle with body image. "My mom was always dieting. My grandparents were always dieting. The mode of choice was 'starve yourself.'" Skinniness and hunger were met with hums of approval by her mother; like the time Quinn commented that so far in that day she had eaten nothing but an apple. Perusing old photos would elicit approving comments like "Look how skinny you were."

Quinn's natural shape never fit neatly into a thin ideal. "I'm very muscular. I've always been. In junior high school, people called me a she-man. I was picked on because I was so much bigger and stronger than many of the boys. It persisted all through high school. I resisted it. I hated how big I was."

Her broad shoulders and powerhouse legs turned out to be a natural fit for rowing, a sport she began participating in at age fourteen. Size classes included a "lightweight" boat; her five-seven frame of 175 pounds made her an unlikely candidate for that one, where female rowers averaged 130 pounds. She asked the coach to let her on, but he refused. "I felt like it would be a good motivator to lose weight—a justification to why I was trying to starve myself."

By the end of high school, she started taking diet pills and laxatives. She remembers being in the car with her boyfriend and having to rush to the bathroom because she'd taken ten laxative pills.

At the end of her junior year in high school, Quinn was raped by a friend of a friend at a house party. This event continued to wreak havoc on her self-image and the trajectory of her life in the years that followed. Although she received scholarship offers from four-year universities to join their rowing teams, she was so traumatized by the experience of the rape that she was unable to focus on schoolwork, friends, or relationships, and certainly not on college admissions. Instead, she chose to attend a small community college so she would be near the home of a close friend.

"I did have feelings of worthlessness," Quinn recalls. "I felt icky. I felt gross."

When she first started going to her local gym, where she discovered mixed martial arts classes, she quickly realized that she loved getting out of her head and into her body. "It was me taking my body back," she explains. "That was the feeling. I could push myself so hard and so much that I didn't have to think about anything else. I could completely be in my body. It was all about what I was doing in that moment. It was amazing to feel that."

She enjoyed meeting the other fighters and learning different forms of mixed martial arts. In the months that followed, she stepped up her visits from twice a week to every day, and particularly enjoyed classes that incorporated weights. Her already athletic physique grew into something more muscular and conditioned. Eventually, the owner and head coach of the facility asked her to coach strength and conditioning classes. The classes would incorporate a CrossFit element, and she was supposed to attend a two-day CrossFit certification course. CrossFit, it turned out, was her jam: She immediately fell in love with it.

"What was so life changing about finding CrossFit was that it didn't matter what you looked like," Quinn points out. "And it was like, for the first time, my body was actually appreciated. People said, 'Wow, you're strong. You push hard.' Here, it was a good thing to walk into the gym and have thick thighs! It was, 'Oh, I bet she can squat a lot of weight.'"

Quinn's relationship with her body changed completely. "All of a sudden my world, my surroundings, were about what my body could do, not a world where skinny was a thing. It was: *Where's the limit of her ability?* and *Is she willing to go find that?* That was life-changing."

She started working as a trainer and over the next decade worked at seven different gyms and entered a dozen different CrossFit events.

"My goal is longevity," Quinn maintains. "I want to be able to wrestle with my grandkids and go hiking in my eighties. I want to live a long, healthy life and be strong." She recounts helping her husband cut and carry sheets of plywood for a home-improvement project. "He was like, 'I am so glad you're strong,'" she says. "*I'm* so glad I'm strong."

The challenge for a lot of women, though, is in holding on to that perspective when all the "get thin" messages are so insistent and omnipresent. Trent Petrie, a professor at the University of North Texas, has spent years studying how female athletes view their bodies and themselves. What he's discovered is that while women athletes have a positive perception of their bodies in the context of their sport and what they are capable of, that gets tested in the real world.

This "duality," Dr. Petrie says, means that body satisfaction derived from what their bodies can *do* doesn't necessarily translate to appearance. "When athletes leave the sports environment and enter the regular environment, they often feel discomfort in their bodies. For a swimmer, that can look like *I love my body when I'm swimming. But when I get out and put my clothes on and I'm meeting someone in a traditional role, I feel awkward, I can't fit into clothes well, I don't look like everyone in the media.*"

His research has helped shed light on an important antidote to this feeling of not fitting in, something called a dissonance-based intervention. This is a tool you can use to actively reject something that might be considered a social norm, through activity, self-convincing, and verbalization. Eric Stice, a professor of psychiatry and behavioral sciences at Stanford who has also utilized the power of this tool to reverse women's disordered body image, calls this a social psychology persuasion principle.

Deploying this powerful tool, Petrie has taken groups of student athletes and gotten them to discuss and critique body pressures together, vocalizing the way these come up in society and addressing them in focus groups. What he's found is that conversation, debate, and imagery—as well as promoting an activist attitude among the women to counteract beauty norms—can have a positive impact on their body perceptions and attitudes. He's also a proponent of the concept of mindful self-compassion, which involves encouraging women athletes to shift how they perceive themselves through a lens of kindness rather than criticism. Finding a sisterhood with other female athletes is key.

Until society consistently drives home the message that women can be powerful and tough—not just thin and delicate—we will have to cultivate that notion for ourselves. But how does one consistently perform that dissonance-based intervention? How do you flip the switch and the script? And perhaps more important, how do you hang on to that message? It requires a change of heart, but also a whole lot of mettle and determination. All of us want to commit to making more nutrient-dense meals or to adhering to a workout schedule for a week. But how do you make it part of your life, part of who you are rather than just something you like to do sometimes? Do you care enough to pack the resistance bands?

I learned about Dr. Stice of Stanford while researching an article. A psychologist, he first became interested in dissonance-based interventions and their potential to help eating disorders as a postdoctoral student at Stanford in 1996, when he saw a patient struggling with anorexia. He recalls spending five sessions trying to convince her to not engage in extreme dieting and not getting anywhere. Then he had an idea. He switched roles with the client, asking *her* to try talking *him* out of having anorexia. He parroted back arguments the client had given him in the past (for example, "Everyone will like me more if I'm thin," or "Clothes look better when I'm thin"), which she had to debunk. The exercise was a powerful one because it forced the client to verbalize arguments against herself in an outward-facing way.

"You could see the gears turning in her head. You could tell attitudes were changing in the session."

Stice tested this technique on more patients and soon realized that such exercises prompt participants to reduce their pursuit of this ideal. Based on this experience, Stice created a dissonance-based eating disorder prevention program called the Body Project, where young women engage in a series of verbal, written, and behavioral exercises to help them debunk their long-held ideal of thinness. For instance, participants discuss societal costs associated with pursuing the thin ideal, complete role plays in which they talk facilitators out of pursuing the thin ideal, and engage in body activism (for instance, placing Post-its saying "You are beautiful—no need to change your appearance" in diet books at a bookstore chain).

"The more you talk with your friends about how much thinner you wish you were and how you're going to lose weight, you are reinforcing that ideal. You are making it stick more deeply in the cranium," Dr. Stice says.

But speaking out about something outwardly also impacts how we feel about it. In other words, by speaking it, you can convince yourself. "We internalize the appearance ideal that has been pushed on us the more we verbally endorse it. So make the time to reject it—that it is not healthy, not working. The social network we choose—our friends and our peers—have a lot of power in reinforcing it or not reinforcing it," he says.

The key, he says, is to outwardly verbalize. "If you're rejecting it in your cranium but not telling everyone else about it, it's not as powerful. By stating it out loud so other people hear it, you become accountable and it's easier to move the attitude."

Stice's work has inspired me. In my mindscape, I make every effort to counteract the formula of "skinny equals success" as part of my own mental hygiene. Because just as society pummels us hard with marketing, why not hit back? I consistently stage dissonance-based interventions: I tell myself, *Skinny's not the solution and strong is beautiful.* I've felt it in my bones as I lift, and make a point of eating plenty of good homemade food. It feels good to nourish my body, care for it, and not feel like I need to be hungry in order to look a certain way.

I find it helpful to *visualize* as well as *verbalize* a strong and healthy body. When preparing food, I say, "I am caring for and nourishing my body." When I see a painfully skinny or obviously photoshopped model, I make an active point of not coveting to look like her, reminding myself, "That's actually an unhealthy and unsustainable level of body fat." I think of it as being a body activist for myself. And I think of the women who came before me, like the Great Sandwina, Charlotte Perkins Gilman, and Pudgy Stockton, who continue to inspire me to buck the norm every single day.

PART TWO

PUSH

Building a Longer Life and Empowering a New Generation

CHAPTER 4

AGING BEASTFULLY

Strength Training for a Longer Life

It wasn't until I was well into my forties that I gave much thought to the aging process. In the last few years, even though my workouts haven't changed, I've felt twinges and aches more acutely than before. My hair has thinned; I've had nights of tossing and turning. I find myself in the throes of perimenopause. As Nora Ephron says, "Anything you think is wrong with your body at the age of 35 you will be nostalgic for at the age of 45."[1]

Weight training has enormous benefits no matter what age we are. And even though the rate at which women gain muscle may slow down a bit as we age, weight training is still effective and important for women in any decade of their lives. It helps combat muscle loss and keeps metabolism and strength up.

Perimenopause and menopause typically hit women from ages forty to fifty-five.[2] In many ways, these are the years when women are at their most vital. By this point, our earning power is hopefully higher than it was when we were younger, and we may have reached a higher level in our profession, or if we have children, they might be entering their late teens or early twenties, becoming independent from us. In a lot of ways, it's our prime.

Most women will live more than one-third of their lives in menopause or postmenopause. More than half of women between fifty and sixty-five say they are the happiest and most fulfilled they've ever been in their lives, according to a Gallup survey once presented at an annual meeting of the North American Menopause Society.[3] It's a time when women are more accepting of their bodies and themselves.

At the age of fifty-three, Myla Bseirani had lived for fifteen years in a deeply unhappy marriage and was navigating a messy divorce. Suddenly, she found herself living alone in Jamesville, New York, with her teenage daughter, Aliya, trying to pay bills on her own as an accountant, barely getting by. The stress was so bad it made her weep, sending her into nightly crying jags. She had little self-confidence, always driven by a feeling that she was "less than."

She'd grown up in the Philippines, immigrating with her parents and two siblings to the United States when she was fourteen. Culturally, where her family came from, women were supposed to suck it up, stay quiet, and accept things, she recalls. Although she didn't know it at the time, she was a fighter.

Myla had a friend from the neighborhood, a carpet installer named Mike Halsey, who had helped her on a home office renovation. Mike was a tall, garrulous guy with a penchant for cursing. He was always tan, fit, and muscular, with a dark mustache and a ready smile. He promoted bodybuilding shows in the upstate New York area and would often "invite" people to compete. It was his corny way of saying hello. "Hey, Mike, when's your next show?" friends would ask. "It's in April. You gonna enter?" he'd ask.

One day in September 2015, just a month after her divorce, Myla was on a long car ride, heading to meet a client in New Jersey. Mike gave her a call—just to check in, as he knew she had been going through a divorce. He mentioned a show he was promoting and did his usual "You gonna enter?" shtick. After telling him to knock it off, Myla drove another hour on the Garden State Parkway, thinking: *Wouldn't it be amazing if I actually entered? Could she change her body and get strong? What if she exercised for a few months and really worked out? What if she used this upcoming show as an excuse to get fit—incredibly fit—and do something she never dreamed possible? Maybe it could be one of those fun, crazy midlife transformations.*

She called Mike back within an hour and said she would compete. She laughs when she remembers how he backtracked: "Well, wait, it's in November, that's eight weeks away, so there may not be enough lead time for you. Did you know there's a whole nutrition element to this? It's not just about exercising." But it was too late. When Myla sets a goal for herself, she doesn't back down. She was determined.

After her conversation with Mike, Myla checked out some books from the library on weight training, one of which was *Weight Training for Dummies*. She bought a few dumbbells from Dick's Sporting Goods—ten, fifteen, twenty, and twenty-five pounds—and spent the next several weeks figuring out how to exercise with them. "I had no idea what I was doing, so I googled everything," she says. "Biceps curls. Triceps extensions. I might have done some lunges."

When she and her daughter walked into that competition at the Landmark Theatre in Syracuse that cold November morning, they immediately felt out of their element. The halls were decked out in banners and photographs of past champions. Coaches and makeup artists trailed behind jacked competitors in spangled-up, colorful bikinis. Myla only had one black backpack filled with her bikini, her clear heels, her stage jewelry, and a pair of flip-flops. Her bikini was simple—a light blue color—purchased from a local seamstress, far less ornate than the elaborate custom jobs that other competitors wore. Shaking with nerves, she stepped out into the bright stage lights, striking her best poses in front of a panel of seven stone-faced judges and managing to place somewhere in the middle. Not the best, not the worst. And certainly not bad for someone who had "winged this thing with a 'For Dummies' book," according to Myla.

The fire had been lit. Those promising results threw fuel on the flames and encouraged Myla to continue on her fitness journey. Over a period of time, she purchased barbells and metal plates—even a circa 1982 leg press machine—so she could expand on her workouts at home. A year later, she joined a gym—Planet Fitness in DeWitt, New York.

Myla's training was a grind. Much of the time she didn't feel pretty and didn't look it, either, grunting and gritting her teeth, sweating through her workout tank tops and leggings. Some days she saw herself in the mirror and thought she looked disheveled and tired. Many days she worked out, not because she desperately wanted to but rather to check a box.

But bit by bit, Myla started to feel better about herself, stronger. Without even realizing it, she was changing her whole way of life. Five months later, she entered another competition, the New York State Natural in Syracuse. This time she felt more prepared; she now knew how to train for optimal physical results and was aware that lean proteins and carbohydrates helped her fill out the muscles on her naturally thin frame. She felt increasingly confident in her ability to pose. She even borrowed a friend's competition bikini, a daring royal blue with rhinestones that captured the light onstage. This time, she came to win.

Two weeks before the competition, however, Myla began feeling pain in her abdomen. After numerous tests and a flurry of doctor's visits, she learned that she had colon cancer. She was crushed, unsure whether to go ahead with competing. But she had put in countless hours at the gym and had completely transformed her approach to nutrition, so she didn't want to give up now. In considerable physical discomfort, Myla decided to delay her cancer treatment by a week in order to compete, continuing to perform her lunges, biceps curls, and squats in the basement every morning in preparation.

When the big day came, Aliya did Myla's hair and makeup and applied her tanning spray before she got onstage, as she still didn't have a coach or a makeup artist. In the bling-covered blue bikini, wearing thick black eyeliner and a fake French manicure, Myla put a huge smile on her face and walked out more confident than ever. She placed first in the contest, earning her the coveted pro status.

A week after the competition, she had her surgery and has since been cancer-free. She's now in a new relationship. Her professional life is flourishing—she owns her own business and works from home—and she considers her fitness lifestyle a pivotal factor in her success. "It gives me a sense of self-worth in everything I approach," she maintains. Myla gets up every day at three a.m.—in pajamas and a sports bra—and heads to her gym setup in the basement. Some days she focuses on legs, other days upper body. Her equipment is simple: barbells, dumbbells, and that clunky metal leg press, and a treadmill for when she needs some cardio. Hitting weights after her first cup of coffee is routine, something she doesn't think about. "It's just like brushing my teeth," she laughs. "I've gained so much confidence from it. Which is huge for me, because all these years I didn't think I could look good or do anything. It's all doable if you're willing to work for it." For her, it's the feel-good aspect of her workouts that keeps her coming back for more. "The 'looks' thing," she explains, "that's just a bonus."

But people do often comment on how much younger she looks, marveling at how she is reversing the aging process. "I'm happier," she explains. "And when you're happier, you look younger. You have more confidence. I mean, yes, I'm in better shape, but I think the confidence is what shows."

Myla's story is a testament to how menopause and aging can be a physically freeing time in our lives. While we're still menstruating, we might have kids we are caring for or careers to which we are intensely devoted. After we stop menstruating, it's as if we're being rewired to take care of ourselves. And, I would argue, this is precisely the time when we can rebuild our bodies, too.

Bodybuilding completely shifted my view of aging. I had once thought that sports were intended for the young. Not shocking, of course, that I or anyone else should have this idea. Sports heroes and the bodies celebrated in advertising all have a youthful aura. Aging bodies certainly didn't read "athletic" to me.

As I learned through competing, bodybuilding is very welcoming to older women of all ages. In most sports, we're told that we peak in our teens and early twenties, but in bodybuilding, there's a concept called muscle maturity. This is an eye-of-the-beholder thing, an aesthetic concept, but the thinking is that muscle maturity occurs only after years of training, and so most women won't achieve it until their thirties and forties. If we look at women bodybuilders on a stage, the older ones clearly have an advantage over the younger. Their bodies are harder, more defined, tougher, and grainier; their muscles are notably more striated. Imagine if the rest of society could look at women's bodies through the lens of bodybuilding, where years and experience are considered an advantage!

Not only do older women have an edge in bodybuilding contests, but the very fact that they are building muscle is giving them an extraordinary protection against the effects of aging on the body. Building muscle counteracts the natural loss of bone density that comes with getting older, and it also reframes the shape of the body into one that looks and actually is younger. If you've ever watched an older woman athlete move, you'll know what I mean. She exudes a distinctive confidence and joy— something in the way she carries herself, in her attitude and her smile. This isn't the result of a cosmetic procedure, a beauty product, a face cream, or an injection. It's as if her discipline and strength can be read in her face and in her movements. She's achieved a greater self-worth: she looks kick-ass and is kick-ass. I feel that sense of self-worth growing in me as well. When I face adversity—rough waters at work, a feud in my family, or some kind of disappointment—I reflect inward and feel my strength. My physical strength holds power, a feeling that I have something that others don't have. It's me. And it's mine.

Bodybuilding for Long-Term Health

In 2017, my coach, Tina Peratino, a forty-four-year-old retired pro bodybuilder blonde whose petite stature belies her tough, authoritative personality, learned that she had lupus, an autoimmune condition that can cause inflammation, joint pain, swelling, and stiffness. No one knows exactly what causes lupus, although it's likely a combination of genetics and environmental factors. Prior to her diagnosis, Tina had been in pain for some time but could never figure out why, chalking it up to her age or to her years of overtraining. She got surgeries for a torn labrum in her shoulder, a torn biceps, tendon issues. "My left has always been the worst," she explains. "My left hip, left shoulder. I would get surgery, then physical therapy, and it would be like, 'Oh, it's better.' And then it would just pop back up."

Tina is the winner of numerous national bodybuilding competitions, but she had retired from competing in 2012, and through 2016, "I just was never well. I was never sick enough to be *sick*. But there were always issues. Digestive issues. Hormone issues." A blood-work panel finally came back showing that Tina had lupus.

"It didn't really change anything, but at least it gave me an answer," she says. "There was a bit of a grieving process. The reality hit me that this was a disease that I was going to have for the rest of my life."

Over time, Tina learned to shift from an unforgiving all-or-nothing mindset to one of continuous training, allowing herself to let it take whatever shape felt possible at a given time in order to keep things moving. One of the most important things I've learned from Tina is that it's possible to be tough and have high expectations for yourself, but also to allow yourself the grace of not getting it 100 percent right all the time. It's okay not to be perfect as long as you keep moving.

After her diagnosis, Tina was determined not to let health challenges keep her from her commitment to staying strong. "Perseverance and resilience are so ingrained in me. There's not a giving-up option." Although she can no longer train at full capacity, she tries to do something active every day, ideally strength based. At least three times a week, she aims to do some kind of full-body circuit for thirty minutes. She usually works out in her garage first thing in the morning. "I go in there and decide what feels good, and I spend about an hour," she says. That might mean tire flips, tire slams (where she bangs the tire repeatedly with a sledgehammer, a great full body exercise), or a "bear complex," where she takes a lightly loaded barbell and completes five repetitions of five exercises—without ever lowering the bar.

"Just staying active is my number one thing," she describes. "If I can't do anything, I get my steps in." At a bare minimum, she'll do 10,000 steps a day. Sometimes she gets on her spin bike for twenty minutes, and if that is all she's able to do, that's fine.

At one time her identity was so completely steeped in body-building that when it went away, she struggled with depression, asking herself, "*If I can't compete, then who am I? What is the point?* I had put so much of myself into that.

"Once I realized it was not so much about winning but about overcoming and pushing forward," she says, things became much easier. "I may not be able to do things the way I want to, but I can do some things. Many things."

She says her years of strength training developed a foundation for both her physical strength and her mental strength. And that it has helped her approach her fifties with a chronic disease head on.

It's never too soon or too late to start building muscle. As women and men age, our muscles shrink, starting in our thirties and progressing more rapidly as we get older. Sarcopenia is the medical name for the age-related loss of muscle mass and strength: We lose some amount of muscle mass per decade as we age, and this becomes a factor in how frail our bodies are and increases the likelihood of falls and fractures. A 2015 report from the American Society for Bone and Mineral Research found that people with sarcopenia had 2.3 times the risk of a fracture from a fall, such as a broken hip, collarbone, leg, arm, or wrist.[4] "Consider it the gray hairs of the musculoskeletal system," says Cheri Blauwet, a sports medicine physician at Harvard who specializes in female masters' athletes, who are typically over age thirty-five.

Here are five ways that strength training can help with things that typically happen in women's bodies as a result of aging, and how it can help counteract the effects of time and promote a stronger life.

1. Stimulating Satellite Cells

Satellite cells are the stem cells responsible for regenerating muscle tissue. (They are called *satellite cells* because of their position orbiting the muscle fiber.) These cells respond to stresses such as injury or exercise by stimulating muscle growth. Estrogen levels have been shown to play a role in the maintenance of these cells, and as estrogen levels decline during perimenopause and menopause, so do satellite cells. Strength training, by contrast, actually helps stimulate these muscle-regenerating cells. In a study where muscle biopsies were taken among over one hundred subjects of different ages, certain types of muscle fibers got significantly smaller with age, accompanied by a reduction in their satellite cell content. Results from a subgroup of older adults in their sixties and seventies who performed twelve weeks of supervised resistance-type exercise training showed that the extra training significantly increased the type II muscle fiber size and satellite cell content in their bodies. If muscular atrophy is a sign of aging, then strength training is a key way to make your body look and feel younger.[5]

2. Building Better Bones

Resistance training helps build bones. Up to 20 percent of a woman's bone density loss happens during the menopausal transition.[6] This is a big deal because bone loss leads to bone fractures, which can significantly reduce quality of life, decrease mobility, cause pain, and increase mortality.

Strength-training activities, as well as weight-bearing aerobic exercises like walking, running, and cycling—activities that place stress on bones—work to build stronger bone matter. While you are exercising, the bones are stimulated to produce more bone tissue—they become denser, so the risk of osteoporosis and fractures decreases.[7] It's a bit like pruning a shrub to encourage it to add growth and look bushier. Activities that put stress on bones stimulate extra deposits of calcium and nudge bone-forming cells into action. The tugging and pushing on bone that occur during strength training in particular provide the stress, which improves the quality of the bone matter.[8]

Even weight-bearing aerobic exercise, like walking or running, can help your bones, but there are a couple of caveats. Generally, higher impact activities such as running, hiking, tennis, climbing stairs, and jumping rope have a more pronounced effect on bone than lower impact aerobics. And keep in mind that only those bones that bear the load of the exercise will benefit. For example, walking or running protects only the bones in your lower body, including your hips.

Weight-bearing exercise can mean exercises that use your own body weight, too—not necessarily just those with equipment such as weights or machines. The key is to keep the activity challenging, says lead researcher and kinesiology scientist Larry Tucker at Brigham Young University. If someone is a regular walker, then just walking probably won't help improve bone density. But incorporating elevation or jump-roping along with other challenges to the regimen will help. "If you're always doing exactly the same thing and never increase the workload, you won't improve," Tucker says in an interview. "Bone is a lot like muscle—it responds to the strains placed upon it."[9]

In a study Tucker conducted that was published in the *Ameri-*

can Journal of Health Promotion, sixty women ages twenty-five to fifty were split into three groups. The first group did light stretching only; the second group performed ten jumps with thirty seconds in between jumps twice daily; and the third group performed twenty jumps in a similar fashion. After sixteen weeks, the women's measured hip bone mineral density was significantly greater in the jumping groups than in the control group.[10]

Strength training in particular targets the bones of the hips and spine, which are among the sites most likely to fracture because they are weight-bearing bones. Workouts that emphasize balance and stability—side lunges, squatting on one leg, reaching and balancing poses—can also help train against falls.

Fractures—particularly ones involving the hip—are a big deal as we age. They are associated with a heightened risk of mortality, particularly within the first year after the fracture took place. In one study, one in eleven women died following a non-hip fracture, increasing to one in five women following a hip fracture.[11]

3. Boosting Metabolism

As levels of estrogen and progesterone lower during perimenopause and menopause, there is a slowing down of metabolism. The upshot is a decrease in muscle mass, resulting in fewer calories being burned. (While muscle doesn't directly burn fat, the more muscle mass you have, the higher your resting metabolic rate.) This means that—without any further exercising—women with more muscle typically burn more calories throughout the day.

"When you are strength training, you are structuring a bigger engine for burning fat," explains Edward Laskowski at the Mayo Clinic. "It's like building a V8 engine instead of a four-cylinder engine."[12]

The muscle tone lost from reduced hormone production is often replaced by fat—and a common settling area tends to be (no surprise) in the midsection. Strength training not only increases calorie burn but also helps us develop better engines for that burning to continue even after we put our weights down.[13]

4. Promoting Better Sleep

About half of women report trouble sleeping during perimenopause, compared with 42 percent before the menopausal transition began.[14] Difficulty staying asleep is the most common complaint among women of a certain age, along with waking up too early and frequently getting up to pee (urinary incontinence is another fun symptom). At the root of these problems are changes in hormones. The same fluctuations that cause hot flashes and night sweats also result in our waking up during the night. Even women who don't have hot flashes say their sleep is worse during this phase of life. One potential reason is that the brain becomes more active during sleep, leading to a lighter and lessened quality of sleep. Seasons also play a role: perimenopausal women have more problems sleeping in the summer than in the winter, when they also have more hot flashes and night sweats.[15]

The impact of lousy sleep goes beyond just a poor night's rest. Insufficient sleep can have an adverse effect on all kinds of health conditions, including cardiovascular disease, cognitive impairments, and mental health issues. What's also clear is that exercise can help. According to a 2013 study published in the monthly journal *Sleep*, of 339 women in various stages of menopause, those who had clear commitments to exercise in the five or so years preceding the one-month study showed significantly better sleep than those who didn't.[16] (The exercise modalities in that study were mostly aerobic, says lead researcher Christopher Kline at the University of Pittsburgh.)

More research is being done on the impact of resistance training on sleep. Another study by Iowa State University researchers showed that resistance exercise may be more effective than aerobic exercise for getting better sleep. Study participants who completed sixty minutes of resistance exercise three times a week for a year slept longer and fell asleep faster than participants who did aerobic-only workouts or even a combination of aerobic and resistance exercises for the same amount of time.[17]

In my personal experience, I believe weight training has helped me maintain good sleep throughout my menopausal transition. I also believe firmly in the power of rest days and having a wind-down routine ahead of when my head hits the pillow. I only drink caffeine in the morning, avoiding it later in the day. I always take a bath. And I enjoy a cup of chamomile or peppermint tea before bed.

My reasons for prioritizing sleep are multiple. In addition to the fact that poor sleep can ruin your day, it's also important for the process of muscle growth. During sleep, the body produces human growth hormone (HGH), which is essential for muscle growth and development, repair of muscle fibers, and metabolism. Some studies indicate that a lack of sleep can decrease protein synthesis, potentially contributing to the loss of muscle mass and function.[18] The right amount of sleep can vary from person to person, but the Centers for Disease Control and Prevention (CDC) recommends that adults get at least seven hours each night. (The CDC also says that one in three adults does not get enough sleep.)[19]

5. Improving Brain Health

"Exercise is the most transformative thing you can do for your brain today," says neuroscientist Wendy Suzuki in a 2017 TED Talk, who says to think of working out as a "supercharged 401(k) for your brain."[20] Our brains experience changes during menopause, including drops in gray and white matter, which lead to what many women feel to be cognitive slide, or "brain fog." Research shows that over 60 percent of menopausal women experience these cognitive slips.[21] And while the good news is that these effects are often temporary and that women's brains eventually stabilize, there are steps women can take in the perimenopausal period to lessen the slide—and exercise plays a big part. The reason: You can't engage the body without engaging the mind. We are thinking when we work out—counting reps, self-correcting or tweaking position or posture, and engaging a mind-muscle connection. Exercise even has a meditative effect, and mindfulness is an important way to counter brain fog. A large part of the brain—about 82 percent of total gray matter volume— can stand to benefit from physical activity, according to research.

Exercise has measurable benefits for the brain, including improved focus, memory, and reaction time. Over the long term, regular exercise can even change your brain's physiology, helping produce new brain cells in the hippocampus. In other words, regular exercise has a protective anti-aging effect on the brain, stimulating it to develop a more robust hippocampus and prefrontal cortex, those areas most susceptible to neurodegenerative disease and cognitive declines in aging.[22] And while working out doesn't necessarily mean you can prevent or cure dementia or Alzheimer's disease, it can help delay the symptoms of those diseases.

A 2017 study of more than 5,800 adults ages twenty to eighty-four found that people who ran a minimum of thirty to forty minutes, five days a week, had an almost nine-year advantage in biological aging at the cellular level. That advantage, according to lead researcher Larry Tucker, is related to the length of telomeres, which are the end caps of chromosomes.[23]

"Each time cells divide, telomeres become shorter," Tucker explains. "So telomeres getting shorter over time is one of the best predictors of how old a person is. Chronological age is highly related to the length of telomeres."

But in addition to age, he says, lifestyle also greatly influences the length of telomeres. And Tucker found that physical activity contributes to longer telomeres, while other factors such as obesity and smoking shorten them. The length of telomeres is "excellent in its prediction of what a healthy lifestyle factor is," he says. The fact that regular exercise contributes to longer telomeres also means that it slows down aging.

Strength training releases proteins that generate new connections in the brain, which have a powerful effect on cognitive function, from memory to reaction time. It also stimulates the release of irisin, a hormone that improves cognitive function.

On episode 87 of *Hit Play Not Pause*, neurophysiologist Louisa Nicola says, "You can literally change the function and the structure of your brain by resistance training alone."[24]

So many of us approach exercise as a way to chase thinness or think of athletics as a chapter in our lives when we were young and in school. But by maintaining a commitment to athletics—in whatever form that might be—into our forties, fifties, sixties, and beyond, we're going to be able to hold on to our strength and our youth and measurably improve the quality of our lives. As I wrote this book, I interviewed women of all ages who continued to demonstrate to me the ways strength training boosted their bodies and minds as they got older.

Edith Murway-Traina says it was only at the age of ninety-one, when she began lifting weights, that she felt something new happening in her body. A competitive spirit and a feeling of invincibility would wash over her as she performed her signature deadlift and bench press, under the watchful eyes of her coach, Bill Beekley.

Edith was born on August 8, 1921, in the Bronx. She worked alongside her father, a shipping clerk in New York's Garment District, from the time she was fourteen. She got married at nineteen and bore five children. Her husband Eddie contracted polio at age thirty-two and used a wheelchair until he died at fifty-two. While having her family she worked multiple jobs—from bookkeeping for a gas station to answering phones at an aviation company. And she was a consummate caretaker, tending to a sick husband and to her children.

But there were flickers of a desire for athleticism in her life. As a child she was drawn to physical play, whether it was games of tag or impromptu neighborhood ball games. "I was a tomboy. I played basketball and baseball and those kinds of things," Edith recalls. "If they needed a tenth man on a team, I was the tenth man."

In a lot of ways, she was a prisoner of her time, when women weren't encouraged to participate in sports in any meaningful way. It wasn't until she was in her seventies that she became able to express herself physically. In the late 1970s, she remarried and moved to Tampa, where she got involved in line dancing, attending classes and events and eventually teaching dancing, becoming locally known at recreation facilities and in senior centers.

Then, in 2012, at the age of ninety-one, Edith's friend Carmen asked her to join her for a senior's exercise class. "Carmen dragged me kicking and screaming," Edith recalls. They met trainer Bill Beekley at a Silver Sneakers class at a local rec center, which included about a dozen seniors in their sixties and up. They did seated exercises with dumbbells, and Bill showed them various stability and balance exercises.

"I was enjoying every time I lifted," she recalls. "Accomplishing things I never thought I would be able to . . . I became an athlete."

In the months that followed, about a dozen of the more dedicated members of the group class followed Bill, a nationally competitive powerlifter, to different gyms and county facilities, where their workouts progressed to barbell lifts.

Edith was a standout. "She was the eldest in the group, and when others saw her and how much she enjoyed doing it, it inspired everyone," he says. She blew her coach away with her fearlessness and facility. "She picked up the technique of the lifts quickly," Coach Bill says. "But it was more than that: She's got a mental drive that's exceptional."

Soon enough, Bill started her on the major composite lifts, but with light to little weight on the barbell: bench-pressing twenty-five pounds, deadlifting fifty. "I had never coached seniors," Bill explains. "She was ninety-one when she started. I was really cautious with the weight." In the following month, that number ran up—thirty-five pounds on the bench and seventy pounds in the deadlift. It was already a big improvement, but Beekley knew there was more there. In the following weeks, Edith hit forty on the bench press and one hundred in the deadlift. "That was impressive—ninety-one or not! But she was ninety-one!" Edith entered a meet called Raw Record Breakers in Tampa and nailed a forty-five on the bench press and a deadlift of 110. Although she was annoyed that she was the only competitor in her age group, it was still a personal best for her at that time. She wanted to keep going.

On February 21, 2016, she hit her record: sixty-seven pounds on the bench press and 150 on the deadlift.

"In the senior games realm, for someone in their fifties and sixties, that's very respectable," says Bill. "For someone in their nineties, that's amazing."

"I was ninety-one when I started lifting weights," Edith describes. "I had no idea I could lift 160 pounds. That was beyond my realm of comprehension. I was just helping a friend make her way to do something she didn't feel comfortable going to herself. But I ended up discovering that I was capable of some things I never dreamed of being able to do."

In 2021, the Guinness World Records announced that Edith was the oldest competitive female powerlifter in the world. By the time her story was published in the *Guinness World Records 2022*, Edith had already celebrated her hundredth birthday. Her friends gave her a birthday party. She was a record holder. "It was a pretty awesome way to celebrate a hundred years of life," says her daughter Honey. Edith died a year and a half later on March 7, 2023, shortly after doctors removed a cancerous mass. "She was still pretty strong physically," says Honey. "But surgery like that on someone that's a hundred and one takes its toll." Even though she is no longer here with us, Edith's legacy lives on— inspiring anyone who learns about her story and proving that it's never too late.

In fact, many people don't discover strength training until later in adulthood. Part of it is because of a widely believed notion that children shouldn't do strength training. Avery Faigenbaum, a pediatric exercise scientist and professor at the College of New Jersey, says he has fought this idea about strength training's being bad for children for years, in an interview calling it a "zombie myth" that won't die. He's conducted research and written numerous scientific articles and books on the subject.[25]

"We now encourage children to engage in strength training to increase bone, tendon, and ligament strength," Dr. Faigenbaum says, adding that weak kids become weak adults. A big reason why elementary-school-aged children need to begin doing bodyweight exercises—things like planks, burpees, inchworms, and hip bridges—is because strength, as Faigenbaum explains, is synergistic: The more comfortable and confident children become when exercising, the more motivated they will be in the future to want to do more. And the children who feel behind tend to stay behind. This dynamic exists at every school playground: Kids with more physical strength are the ones hanging on the monkey bars or racing for the next available swing. The weak ones are those seated on the sidelines. The pattern feeds on itself and lasts for many years to come: The stronger kids continue on with sports, their enjoyment builds, and their confidence soars. "It's the stronger kids that continue to climb the ladder," Dr. Faigenbaum says. "Strength is totally foundational, and it's for life."

In a program that he runs in cooperation with New Jersey school systems, he trains boys and girls as young as age seven. "We start with just body-weight exercises—squats and so forth—or very light weights, and kids earn the right to use heavier weights by proving they've mastered proper technique."

There's no doubt that children in the United States and other Western countries are weaker than they have been in the past. They're more sedentary, thanks in part to being easily seduced by ubiquitously available technology, and the consumption of ultra-processed foods continues to grow across segments of the U.S. population. The rate of obesity among youth ages two to nineteen years was 10 percent in the United States between 1988 and 1994; that rose to 18.5 percent in the period between 2015 and 2016, according to the Centers for Disease Control and Prevention.[26]

"Whether you are six or sixty, having strength is absolutely essential to movement—to getting out of a chair or walking up a flight of stairs," Dr. Faigenbaum argues. "It is essential to enjoying life." He recently developed a new curriculum called "Animals in Motion" that makes strength and resistance exercises a part of gym classes in public schools in New Jersey and Pennsylvania. No additional weights are needed; the moves use only body weight and are simple and effective. Through his program, Dr. Faigenbaum has transformed traditional mandatory physical ed exercises into a more accessible and dynamic experience for children. They perform frog jump squats, build core strength with crocodile planks, and work their arms and legs by doing bear crawls, improving their balance, stability, and equilibrium so that they can thrive in other activities as well. As the students use their muscles in new ways, they begin to develop a stronger sense of self and better physical coordination. Older kids in these schools might use lightweight dumbbells and medicine balls, but the objective is to keep things light and fun. "They realize this type of training can be enjoyable," Faigenbaum says. "They like that it's a little bit hard, but they think they can do it. It keeps them engaged and it becomes part of their routine, so that by the time they become teenagers, these long-held myths [about weights stunting children's growth] aren't on their radar."

In a huge step for proponents of strength training, the World Health Organization announced in November 2020 that physical activity for children should include not only sixty minutes per day of moderate to vigorous physical activity but also exercises "that strengthen muscle and bone at least three days a week," such as chin-ups, push-ups, and squats.

In 2001, researchers from the Institute for Women's Health at Texas Woman's University reported in *The Journal of Pediatrics* that adolescent girls who were engaged in resistance training had greater bone density in certain areas than girls in a control group. Greater bone density means a greater ability to withstand loads. And as such, their leg strength was measured to be greater—by 40 percent.[27] But there's another benefit for girls in particular, trainers say. Putting weights in their hands at younger ages and teaching them proper use gives them a sense of self-assurance and presence. Later in the weight room during their teen and adult years, they won't feel like a fish out of water. "They can step in there with confidence and be able to say to someone, 'Hey, I'm using those weights,' without feeling weird," says coach and physical therapist Meghan Wieser, who says she has increasingly been working with girls as young as fourteen years old—something that would have been unheard of earlier in her career.

In fact there are a number of ways our habits influence our young children, who, for better or for worse, mimic us and look up to us. Here are some techniques to set them on the right foot:

1. Lift weights with (or at least alongside) your child.

In my basement gym setup, my youngest daughter will sometimes ask to join me. I'll be completing a set, and she'll ask what the exercise is called and if she can do it, too. She'll do maybe one or two sets and call it a day. And that's totally fine. She is learning the value of building—rather than diminishing—herself. She sees that it takes discipline and day-to-day consistency—traits that are valuable in all kinds of life ventures, from doing schoolwork to staying organized and on task. Whether you have sons or daughters, it's important to teach young people that women and strength go together.

Eleven-year-old Ava Gibson began lifting by watching her mother, Taryn Gibson. Taryn had started taking CrossFit at a local gym in Greenville, South Carolina, while her young daughters, then aged seven and nine, ran around in the background. After the girls told her, "We want to try weightlifting!" and Taryn saw that the gym offered private weightlifting lessons, she enrolled both her daughters—Addie and Ava—to try it out twice a week in the evening.

After a few weeks, Addie switched to gymnastics, but Ava took to weightlifting right away. Team sports—which she had dabbled in during summer camp activities—had never really captivated her. She preferred challenging herself independently.

"Teams always have to work together and be on the same page, which is hard," Ava says. "If you're by yourself, you just kind of roll with it."

Inspired by her daughter, Taryn began taking weightlifting lessons as well, thinking it might help her get better with Cross-Fit, which has weightlifting components built into the workouts. By fall of 2022, Taryn and her daughter Ava were taking lessons together, and before long, they both began competing in weightlifting contests.

Ava likes the discipline. "We don't always max out on how much we can lift. Some weeks we just work on doing it right. Other weeks we work on big weight. But most of the time, when we get it right, we can put on a little weight." It's slow and incremental work, and it feels like a reward when she reaches a new goal. "We don't always get to put, like, five more pounds on."

Ava goes to the Greenville Weightlifting Club with her mother three times a week. The club has a dozen young people ages nine to sixteen taking lessons, and it's become a community for her. She's become especially close friends with a fourteen-year-old girl named Ainsley who comes over to the house for sleepovers, movies, and popcorn—and arm wrestling.

Her mom, who has since purchased the club, says that she believes the sport has shielded her daughter from the body issues that can start to creep in with girls of this age.

"She's very interested in clothes and style, but she's never mentioned 'I look fat' or anything like that. She's more, 'Look at my biceps.'"

2. Own your size. Take up space. Love your body.

Bodybuilding has made me stand up taller and carry myself more broadly. I put a lot of work into my frame, and it's something that has given me confidence in myself. When I'm around my children, I make a habit of only speaking positively about my body and my workouts. And they love that their mom is strong. On one occasion, while I was pulling on jeans that no longer fit, my older daughter said it was probably because of my quad muscles. A previous version of me would have blamed myself for eating too much, but instead, I laughed and loved that she had made that comment. The more positively you speak about your strength and size around kids, the more they will want to emulate your approach.

Chassity Del Balso doesn't remember a time when she wasn't around weights in a gym. The fourteen-year-old's father, CJ, was a high school physical education teacher who helped introduce teenagers at Arnold O. Beckman High School in Irvine, California, to weights during gym class. When the family moved to

Omaha, Nebraska, he opened his own gym, called Conqueror Weightlifting, in a 2,100-square-foot industrial space. His dream was to teach Olympic weightlifting and also introduce young people to the power of strength training to maximize their athletic performance in other youth sports.

"It's one of the most potent things you can do in terms of developing explosiveness, even for an uncoordinated kid. You wield a barbell overhead and that teaches balance, kinesthetic awareness, keeping the movement sharp." But more than that, he says in an interview, it sparks a transformation inside. "You can see it. They walk around taller. It's why I like working with kids."[28]

He's coached football, strength training, and conditioning at the high school level and later specialized in coaching weightlifting and even competed once as an adult.

Chassity watched attentively. One of her earliest memories was seeing her dad win his master's class at the Texas State Weightlifting Meet in San Antonio. "I was four or five years old. I felt really happy and proud of him. I remember seeing his face, smiling." She keeps a photograph of that moment tucked away in her night table.

CJ began teaching Chassity technique when she was eight years old. He would place a five-foot-long PVC pipe in her hands and show her how to squat with it in the garage at home. It came naturally to her. "She was abnormally good," he recalls. Chassity eventually came into the gym and worked on the floor, alongside adults, two times a week. "I taught her like anyone else, but with lighter weights."

At eight years old, Chassity competed in her first competition, followed by more than two dozen meets since then. She has won national championships in her age and weight category. She now works out at the gym for about an hour and a half four times a week—and has taken on other sports, from track and field to tae kwon do.

But the gym, near her father and other weightlifters, is her favorite place. "I like seeing people happy and how strong they can be. There's kindness in the gym. And discipline," she says.

It's a great example of the power we have as parents to model strength—and the mighty power of harnessing, valuing, and building it—to our children. CJ's wife, LaShanda, also runs and lifts weights several times a week. "Chassity's never not been around it, all around her, and I think seeing it that way helps."

What's remarkable about these girls is that they are actively avoiding and even disrupting the messages that tend to hit young women when they reach puberty: that it's more important to fit in, to be nice, and to take up as little space as possible. Boys are more often praised for leading, but girls are taught to fear it, worried that they might get made fun of or become ostracized. In a study by the Girl Scout Research Institute, a third of girls who said they do not want to be leaders said they felt that way due to a fear of being laughed at, of making people mad at them, of coming across as bossy, or of not being liked by people.[29] Girls still grapple with trying to adhere to stereotypical "feminine" behaviors such as getting along with everyone, being nice, and appearing easy to please.

Between elementary school and high school, girls' self-confidence drops sharply. Girls tend to deflect praise and minimize their achievements. They grow up to become women who wait to apply for a job until they meet 100 percent of the criteria, versus 60 percent of men who typically do, according to an often-cited statistic from Hewlett Packard.[30] But being involved in a practice that builds your body and forces you to lift heavy things over your head seems to be doing something to these girls' sense of what their capacity is and where their limits lie. And my sense from speaking with them is that they are brimming with confidence and able to meet and push through their goals. Chassity says that when boys in her class make derogatory comments about her size, she easily brushes them off. "They just don't understand," she explains.

3. Enjoy your food.

It's time to quit the negative self-talk around food. Instead of sending your child the message that food is something to be restricted and avoided, instead encourage good eating habits by eating well and talking in terms of how good it feels when you eat. Try saying things like "Wow, that was really nourishing!" or "I love all these colors on the plate!" Avoid "Ugh, that made me feel bloated!" Or "I love that—but so many calories!" As women, we've often overheard and repeated phrases without thinking, but our children take note. They also watch our behavior. We must break the cycle. Child psychologists say this is the number one way we can stop disordered eating dead in its tracks and improve kids' body image.

4. Brag. Shine. Own your successes and strengths.

Women are conditioned to downplay their successes and accomplishments, and female confidence is often taken for arrogance. A recent study coauthored by researchers at Harvard

Business School and the Wharton School of the University of Pennsylvania asked nine hundred participants to take a twenty-question test and to guess their score. On average, the women reported their performance to be fifteen points lower than the average man. That's even though women and men, on average, performed equally well on the test.[31]

In the case of young Bronwyn Aldrich, strength training encouraged her to unapologetically own the idea that she could push, pull, and lift heavy things, taking pleasure once in showing a group of boys playing by the river how she could lift a heavy rock just like them, her mother recalls. At twelve years old, Bronwyn was done with ballet and started taking up weightlifting after watching her mother take classes. Since then, lifting has added a new element to her confidence.

Bronwyn says that she enjoyed the fact that the improvements she made—in lifting more weight—were measurable over time. And so she increased her training to three days per week from two. And her body started to transform from that of a lithe child ballet dancer to a more athletic and broad-backed tween. Bronwyn has a twin sister, Aeralind, who is also a ballet dancer. And her mother, Melissa, has noticed an uptick in confidence in the way Bronwyn talks about herself. At the beginning of the pandemic, their mother says, both girls looked identical. But now Bronwyn weighs 118 to Aeralind's 108 pounds. Her back is visibly broader. And she generally wears a size or two up in pants. "She loves being strong," says Melissa. "She'll brag to her sister, 'I weigh more than you! And it's all muscle.'"

Years ago, as a young reporter in my twenties, I had the privilege of sitting next to a more senior female colleague and got to hear the way she worked. She always made a point to tell new sources she called about her most recent stories, expecting them to have read or know about them. The tactic had a not-so-subtle "Do you know who I am?" vibe. I later became friends with my now semi-retired colleague Joann Lublin, and have long admired her, but my inexperienced self thought she was really full of herself and liked to brag. Now I look back and realize that if she had been a man, I would have just considered him assertive and confident. And while it's taken me many years, I have recently begun introducing myself on the phone with new sources utilizing the same brag-sheet tactic. It's a little daily moment of standing up for myself in a public-facing way—and I always think of her with gratitude.

5. Get your child involved, not just in strength training, but in sports of all kinds.

Discovering role models is important, and sport is a way for children to find their superheroes. It's also an ecosystem in which they learn important life skills such as teamwork, leadership, aggression, and communication, as well as shaking hands after a crushing loss and getting back up when they fall down. It can teach you to finish the job and rise above challenges—even when things aren't working out the way you'd like. A 2018 study conducted by Ernst & Young found that 94 percent of women who hold C-suite positions are former athletes.[32]

6. Put your oxygen mask on first.

Studies show children feel better when they see their parents taking care of themselves. Ellen Galinsky, president and cofounder of the Families and Work Institute, conducted a nationally representative study back in the late 1990s—whose centerpiece was a survey of 1,023 children ages eight to eighteen—that became the foundation of her book *Ask the Children: The Breakthrough Study That Reveals How to Succeed at Work and Parenting*. Galinsky said parents were surprised to learn that their children weren't necessarily craving more time with them. If given "one wish" to improve how their parents' work affected them, the largest proportion of children wished their parents were less tired and stressed, rather than wanting more time with them.[33] It's time we put away our guilt and start thinking about the incredible lessons we can teach our daughters—and sons—by making time for rest and building self-care into our lives.

PART THREE

LIFT

Taking Our Bodies Back

CHAPTER 5

THE MENTAL GAME

Don't Overthink and Find Your Why

Getting Into the Mindset

Hopefully by now, you're intrigued enough by lifting weights and strength training that you're considering incorporating them into your routine. Or maybe you've already added strength training and weights into your life and you want to know how to take it to the next level. Where do you start, and how do you get to where you need to go? The first and most important thing you can do is to shift your mindset. Bodybuilding for me isn't just about the muscles. I mean, I like the muscles, but it's more than that—it's about being in the zone. It's the zeroed-in lifestyle choice that has me hooked, being in a completely focused state, day-to-day, when it comes to all things food and exercise—despite whatever else is going on in life. This laser-like focus is really the essence of the sport. In contrast to the flashiness of the competition stage, the day-to-day training involves slurping egg whites on the go or packing ziplocked chicken boob in a purse and then avoiding a post-workout disheveled appearance on a Zoom call. In addition to the complete and total devotion to strength training and weightlifting at least four times a week, there's the relentless daily attention to what I eat: chopping and boiling, measuring, weighing, tracking my intake to ensure there's always a precise balance of macronutrients and micronutrients, packing portions to take to work or on trips, taking supplements, avoiding restaurants, and always planning ahead. The name of the game is commitment.

Mindset is as intrinsically important as physical capability for any athlete. According to Idan Ravin, an athletic performance specialist who has trained NBA All-Stars, including Stephen Curry and Kevin Durant, there are certain mindset traits that distinguish top sportspeople, and some of these traits can even eclipse natural talent or genetic disposition, becoming a more important driver of success. Here are the most critical ones, according to Ravin:

Persistence: There's a day in, day out quality to training that can become very difficult to hit on certain days. Sure, everyone can hit it once in a while, but nailing it consistently is where the needle really moves. And it's hard to get there because . . . life. Other needs become pressing. We get tired. Sometimes we just don't feel like it. But the thing that distinguishes those who succeed is their persistence: Athletes who succeed care. "They really, really care. They care deeply," says Ravin. Although it's tough, make the commitment to a lifestyle that involves hitting a workout on most days—some kind of workout—and prepping meals at the front end of the week. Be all in. Be precise and unyielding: This is training for life—just as valid as training for an event. And if a full workout is too much, I'm of the belief that something is always better than nothing. A long walk, or a fifteen-minute active stretch routine before taking a bath in the evening? That's way better than diving into chips, beer, and a movie and then conking out.

Objectivity: Sometimes we make excuses. "The best athletes play it straight with themselves when they fail. They know it and they expect better," says Ravin. Be honest with yourself. Are you taking care of yourself? Are you giving it what you can? Are you looking for an easy way out? Take stock of the week. What are you doing well? What do you need to do better? It's okay to be hard on yourself when you need to be. Don't be afraid to demand more, whether it's being consistent or getting more organized or prioritizing.

Resilience: It's easy to fall into the all-or-nothing trap. When we slip, we give up and quit the game plan entirely. Don't worry about misses: missed opportunities, missed workout days, mishaps with food. Don't get lost in obsessing. Just keep getting up and moving forward.

The mental and the physical are so deeply intertwined: you can't have the physical piece without the mental. I call the moment when the two converge in an unshakable pact to change habits the fuck-it moment. It manifests itself as an ability to step outside of myself and see how easy it would be *not* to do the hard thing, whether that's the better food choice or the trip to the gym or the run in the rain. I see that my body wants to give up. But it's an inherent knowing that I can and will get it done, this getting uncomfortable. And that by doing so, I will accomplish something better for myself—something that maybe I can't see right now, but I will see in the long run.

When I spoke with forty-six-year-old Donnajeanne Liu-Young, she told me she had competed in nearly a dozen meets since she began training in weightlifting seven years ago. Growing up in Fort Washington, Maryland, the youngest daughter of immigrant parents from the Philippines, she dutifully went to ballet classes three times a week, took piano lessons, and participated in beauty pageants, eventually attending the University of Maryland. "They [her parents] were supportive whenever my interests were in activities that seemed more feminine."

But in her twenties she discovered rock climbing, joining friends several times a week at a climbing gym in an activity that became a physically active version of a happy hour gathering. She found she relished the challenge. After a few years, a different group of friends invited her to join them at CrossFit, and she began attending classes on alternating days with rock climbing. CrossFit opened her up to an athletic lifestyle along with a friendly yet competitive community where she felt at home. She eventually decided she enjoyed CrossFit more and did it exclusively.

In the past, Donna had put a lot of her focus on losing weight, obsessively checking the scales. "CrossFit really opened my eyes to not think about what the 'norm' is. My mindset changed from 'I want to lose weight' to 'Actually, I don't care about how much I weigh. I want to do better in hitting this goal or that time.'"

It was the strength aspect that drew Donna to CrossFit, and she enjoyed the feeling of gaining confidence and strength. Week after week, she was able to put on more plates and lift more weight. "I liked the barbell and strength-training aspect of CrossFit the most," she explains. She learned Olympic weight-lifting, a particular style of lifting weights focused on both the technical movement and the sheer power of lifting weight over-head. Her specialties became the clean and jerk and the snatch, the movement of sweeping a barbell overhead, combining a quick deftness with a big, superhero quality.

Over time, her body changed, becoming tighter and more muscular. Her clothes fit better. She had more energy and confidence. The changes weren't reflected in her weight, but she didn't mind. "I was less concerned with the number on the scale when I had this capability to do these big lifts."

Donna entered her first weightlifting competition in 2018. She joined a weightlifting club, began coaching at the club, and entered a half-dozen competitions in the years that followed. She also became a nationally sanctioned official with the sport's governing organization. She enjoys being a sounding board to the club's members, over half of whom are women, particularly when issues about body image come up. "We're all different sizes and shapes," she points out. "All that matters on the platform is how much you can lift overall. Look at your progress from where you started and where you are today. And you look at your goals. I completely shifted the focus from appearance to performance."

Setting Boundaries and Being Prepared for Fit-Shaming

In the weeks after I had come home from my first competition, I attended a family gathering. Most of the relatives who were there acknowledged my experience, some congratulating me on my ranking and others mentioning that they enjoyed reading my article. But I noticed that one family member in particular, someone I'd been close with growing up and had been excited to see at this reunion, steered clear—of me and of any conversation related to me or my accomplishment. Was it discomfort with the concept of female strength? A judginess about a sport that ranks women based on appearance? Her behavior was difficult to ignore, and I left the gathering feeling hurt and confused.

The disappointing incident with my family was not unique; everyone on a journey to health will encounter judginess. It is one of the most potent roadblocks you're going to face. The biggest influence on your commitment is going to be those around you—friends, family, acquaintances, colleagues. It's best to not expect everyone to be supportive—at least not all the time. Sometimes a lifestyle involving strength and commitment doesn't fit into the way that people perceive women and what they "should" be doing. Perhaps my judgy family member would have been more comfortable with my striving for a skinny figure, taking care of others, or neglecting to make time for myself! In the same vein, you might encounter eye rolls and snarky comments. You might experience jealousy and snide remarks. Friends might say things like "I wish I had that kind of commitment" or "I don't have that kind of time."

Sometimes you'll experience a real pressure to make others feel more comfortable, especially at gatherings, where a well-meaning friend or relative may want to share a bottle of wine or a slice of cake. Food and alcohol are part of the culture and inform the way we socialize, celebrate, and even bond with one another.

This kind of fit-shaming is real, and it can be a serious obstacle to the pursuit of your goals. Fitness and nutrition coach Allison Fahrenbach says she often hears about it through her clients who are trying to focus on a plan and be disciplined, but who have to put up with remarks from friends and family who want to offer their own bit of pseudoscience ("Plant-based is better for you") or comment on appearance ("Are you trying to lose weight?"). It can get tiring. Allison advises to simply focus on yourself and recognize that your new lifestyle can make those around you feel guilty. That in turn can lead to the kind of negative commentary that can be unpleasant. "If your friends or co-workers are eating poorly and you're not, it can cause them to reflect on their own choices," says Allison. By making jabs at you and trying to get you to indulge alongside them, the haters somehow feel better, but it can easily derail your efforts if you're not careful.

The point of all this is that your health, wellness, and fitness are a form of pact with yourself, and they are really nobody else's business. It's important to set boundaries. It's okay to say no to a second helping of dinner, a glass of wine, or a plate of dessert, especially when you're working to meet personal health and fitness goals. Everyone has an opinion on what to eat and how and whether they should exercise. You will likely get a reaction from someone when it comes up. Be ready.

The fact remains, it's really hard not to care about what others think, especially for people pleasers, who enjoy making others feel happy. Navigating a changing body and mindset and the re-action of others to these can be especially tough for women.

Maggie Francis, a graduate student in psychology, was twenty-seven when she says the issue of her physique came up in her relationship with her boyfriend, Johnny.*

Maggie and Johnny were bench pressing at the gym together when she attained a personal best. "I hit 135 pounds, then my goal of 145," she recalls. She had been stuck at lifting 135 pounds for some time but was feeling good that day, and Johnny's pres-ence helped boost her confidence. Gulping down some water, Maggie took a happy sweaty selfie with her iPhone. But any sense of joy or pride was eroded when suddenly Johnny inter-jected: "Don't post that on Instagram."

He appeared uncomfortable, and she encouraged him to tell her why. In the year since they began dating, he said, Maggie had gotten more muscular. He began scrolling through pictures of the two of them on his phone, to make his case. Maggie didn't argue: "It's true, I did change," she says, noting that she now weighs more than her boyfriend. "I'm 175 pounds, he's 135."

She had noticed in recent weeks that Johnny's friends would make jabs about "the girlfriend," often couched as jokes: "Is she going to carry you upstairs?" or "She's stronger than you, bro." He would wince noticeably in response.

In the days that followed the selfie incident, Johnny, who didn't have the healthiest habits generally, started to step up his workouts and pay more attention to his diet. But it didn't last long.

---

* Name changed to protect the identity of the individual.

Soon he reverted back to his old ways, while making cutting re-marks about Maggie's workouts, calling her commitment to her fitness routine "obsessive." Maggie began to question the rela-tionship and his support. "You're making me feel bad for being an athlete," she stated flatly one morning after breakfast.

The reality was that Maggie had struggled with her body im-age for most of her life, starting in middle school, where the skinny popular girls made her feel insecure about her body. In eighth grade, she began restricting her food, as she says, "to stay within the acceptable social range of thinness." She remembers googling information about breast implants in the ninth grade and eating so little she would often feel hungry.

By then, Maggie was a star athlete in track and field and cross-country, with a strikingly powerful physique; she had ripped shoulders and biceps, and her quad muscles showed impres-sively through her shorts and leggings. Her athletic build en-abled her to perform at her peak. But when she was a sophomore in college, her cross-country coach told her she was fat. "My girls don't have love handles," he scolded, adding that she needed to lose weight in order to run faster.

Maggie was devastated, but she also didn't know any better than to agree with him. Her favorite stars those days included Paris Hilton and Kate Moss, and she loved watching *America's Next Top Model*; admiring the long, lean body types on television "made all of it worse."

"My whole life I wanted to be super skinny," she reflects. "I hated my legs because they're big."

It wasn't until she entered a gym as a graduate student in her late twenties and encountered a group of women lifting weights and entering fitness competitions regularly that she felt like she had come home. The women looked strong and confident.

"They intimidated men," she laughs. "I wanted that."

Now she was dating someone who clearly felt intimidated by *her*. Maggie started wearing long sleeves when she was out with Johnny—to cover her muscular arms so that he would be more comfortable—but she didn't like how the tops made her look, and she didn't appreciate having to hide the impressive results of her hard work.

Today, after four years of consistently rigorous workouts, balanced nutrition, and deep introspection, Maggie loves her muscles and feels that she gets respected more now that she has them. But there are those like her boyfriend who aren't used to seeing strong female bodies. When I first spoke to Maggie for this book, her relationship with Johnny was at a standstill. "It's something we're still struggling with," she said. (In a later interview, she said the two had since broken up.)

Rather than letting her boyfriend diminish her self-confidence or discourage her from her fitness goals, however, Maggie came up with an antidote. She started spending more time with people who do encourage her—friends from the gym, family members who want her to be happy and healthy, and colleagues who commend her work ethic. She has since competed multiple times in multiple bodybuilding federations. She even ditched a coach who she felt pressured her to take performance-enhancing drugs. Her sport has helped her be strong in her body as well as in her mind, fueling a confident, can-do ethic.

Here are some tips to help you shift your mindset, stay on track, and drown out the naysayers:

1. Surround yourself with yay-sayers.

There's a lot involved in the way we see our bodies: how we view our desirability and sexuality, how we value ourselves, how we want to be perceived. Just as you physically build your body, your feelings about your body may also be a work in progress. There have been and always will be external pressures and expectations. If the challenge was only what's presented in magazines and on packages, that would be easy. But the really hard stuff lies in what you *think* the people closest to you want you to look like—and how to buck those expectations to forge your own path, staying the course, narrowing the focus to yourself and your own goals.

One of the biggest boosts you can give yourself while going through a major physical and mental transition is to do exactly what Maggie has been doing: surround yourself with people who support you and are rooting for you. Studies show that positive peer influences can have a strong effect on fitness. Research from Vanderbilt University published in the journal *Pediatrics* covered networks of friends in after-school programs involving students ages five to twelve.[1] The researchers tracked kids' physical activity levels over twelve weeks. During the period the children spent in the program, the strongest factor influencing how much time they spent engaged in physical exercise was the activity level of their four to six closest friends. In fact, children changed their exercise level about 10 percent or more to better match those in their circle; children who hung out with more active students were more likely to increase their physical activity levels, while those who befriended more sedentary children became less active. As the study suggests, when you have people close to you who are active, you're likely to become more active.

2. Find communities outside of immediate friends and family if necessary.

Fitness requires dedication and consistency, and when you're not keeping company with those who share your commitment, this can really hinder your progress. If you don't have folks in your immediate friendship group or family who want to support you, you can still find supportive communities. Facebook has thousands of groups for women in fitness, and even if you don't join one of them, you can still follow good role models on Instagram or TikTok. There are so many options now due to social media and streaming, a whole host of ways to surround yourself with women in athletics and positive messaging. Of course, local gyms and even online classes are also places to find like-minded people.

You don't have to feel like you're doing this alone. Working out with others who share your mindset is so affirming. As the internet meme goes, fitness isn't something you do, it's something you are. And when we surround ourselves with messages of athleticism—even if we have to seek them, and they are not always there—it's easier to stick to our goals and withstand fit-shaming. Your mantra should be: "This is who I am. This is the lifestyle I have chosen."

3. Remind yourself that it's okay to be selfish, and that when others make comments, it says more about them than you.

When I find myself experiencing judgment or negativity from others, I remind myself that I'm not doing this for them; I'm doing it for me. Training is an inherently selfish pursuit, and I find it helpful to really indulge in that part of it. In this way, I can focus on what I want to do rather than on what people are saying.

Just do you. Be responsible to yourself, but let nobody meddle in what you eat, how you exercise, or how you live your life. If strong scares them, that's their problem. I also remind myself to give the naysayers the benefit of the doubt: "My grandmother trying to feed me lasagna isn't actually trying to sabotage my new diet; she's just showing me that she loves me."

4. Establish your goal and write it down.

If we're honest, part of caring about our appearance involves caring about what other people think. After all, we want others to think we look good. That's why you must set a goal, blocking out the noise or anything else that seems to get in the way. The first step is to establish a clear and precise goal—a mission statement, if you will. I like to write it down. Some possible goals might be to lift a certain number of pounds, to walk every single day, or to enter a competition. Make your goal clear and positive, something you own that's for you and nobody else. Your goal will likely change over time, but that's okay, too. Weight loss might be part of the goal. That's fine. Just don't treat it as the central do-or-die thing. Don't make your journey all about hitting a number on the scale. Once you have your goal written down, put it in a place where you see it all the time. Tape it to the wall or the fridge. Notice it. Honor it. And then set a time frame during which you are willing to commit to the work to achieve it.

5. Find a structure and rhythm for your training that works for you.

While some people value the ability to adjust their workout schedule based on other moving pieces in their lives, others do better with structure and like to train at a certain time. "I tend to advocate for the latter," says fitness and nutrition coach Allison Fahrenbach. She believes that the body starts to anticipate the workout, in the same way it does for eating and sleeping routines. Exercise, eating, and sleeping tend to work in harmony—a good workout gives you an appetite and can help lead to a restful night's sleep.

Plenty of women I know like to get their workout over with first thing in the morning. For me, I like to exercise in the late afternoon, sort of as a clear-my-head study break. I like to have the freedom of being flexible on timing. I like music. If I'm working out at home in the basement, I physically close the door. I set an intention. I signal to others in my family that this is my time, my space—what I need for my batteries to work. If my kids are home, I'll put a Mommy's Workout sign on the door and tell them to come bug me only if they really, really can't hold out for forty-five minutes. It usually works, but most important, it signals to everyone in the family that this is a vital part of my life. Other times, I'll allow my kids to participate and let the workout become a playful thing, something to experience together: I've used my younger daughter as a bouncy weight for hip thrusts, which makes her burst out laughing. Or we toss a medicine ball or do some yoga stretches. I'll also introduce my older daughter to some lifts, using very small amounts of weight (or even just her body weight).

Lately, I have enjoyed the rhythm of bringing my laptop to the gym, working from a quiet corner of a café space there and then getting one or two workouts in as my study break. It can be a powerful no-excuses way to make fitness a part of the day. After all, you're already at the gym. (And gyms, taking advantage of so much empty office space, are expanding and offering co-working spaces, sometimes for an extra fee.)

6. Find your why.

In my experience, a goal isn't really about looking a certain way for a photo shoot or a wedding. It's about what's really driving that. Is it commitment? Desire? Discipline? Reconnecting with your lost inner athlete? Find that feeling—the why—and write it down alongside your goal. Put it on a sticky note or an index card and tape it to your mirror or your desk alongside your goal. And plunk the words *my why* in there, to formalize and name it.

7. Commit to two lifestyle changes at first.

In order to make progress toward your goal, commit to two lifestyle changes: one involving food, the other involving exercise. For example, you might choose to track your food, writing down what you consume and when you eat it. Do this without judgment; it can be a useful exercise just to see what your rhythms tend to be. Or maybe it's switching out alcohol for seltzer, tea, or kombucha for the next three months. Or if you have a penchant for hitting sweets after a certain hour in the evening, try an evening "shutdown" of the fridge. Just have herbal tea or water after dinnertime, and maybe some carrot and celery sticks if you need to munch on something. But commit to what will be better for your body.

Don't expect your mind to jump directly from square one to square ten. That will set you up for discouragement. Take things slowly. Commit to exercising three days a week. Think about what kind of exercise you enjoy. Is it walks? Jogs? Stretching? Try to incorporate weights into your routine. Perhaps strap on ankle weights or a weighted vest during your walks or employ some dumbbells to add juice to a floor stretch.

As that starts to feel good, you can begin to explore other approaches. Maybe it's the use of some weight-bearing machines at a local gym for two of those days, an exercise class on another day, and brisk walks for one or two days in the week. Or find a way to incorporate exercise into your social life. (I've tried to include something that takes me out of my comfort zone at least once a week. I've taken up tennis and golf.)

8. Exercise is self-care—claim this for yourself.

Exercise isn't just a treadmill. It's not something women should do because they feel guilty about eating something rich or want to reduce a number on the scale. I used to work out for vanity. But now I do it because it's a way of life. It's my form of self-care. And I owe it to myself to do something a little bit uncomfortable each day. It's what makes me feel alive. It feels good to go and move your body and not let life get in the way. I turn off my phone for an hour and lift. Everything else can wait. Self-care doesn't have to mean manicures and massages. "I put it all on the bar," champion powerlifter Tricia Floyd says of the way she approaches her daily lifting sessions. This is a physical metaphor for the way she lifts away her problems, hang-ups, and dilemmas. It is a mindset that she says not only challenges her physically but has also shifted the way she tackles every hurdle in her life.

CHAPTER 6

BUILDING YOUR ROUTINE

A Guide to Beasting Out

Around three o'clock in the afternoon, every afternoon, I take a break from work. This might be a coffee break to anyone else, but it is my time to beast out. I put on music and start with a little warm-up: a few minutes of boxing jabs, some spins on the stationary bike, some jumping rope, or a jog around the neighborhood. I do some stretches. If it's cold outside and I can access a gym with a sauna, I go in there to stretch and get warm. I don't look at any of this as an obligation. This is a treat. It is one of the best parts of my day—intimate and important—because it's truly mine. It's happily selfish—all about me, my self-worth, my value, and my strength. How many other times in the day do we get the opportunity to center ourselves in this way? Normally, I break out either late morning or late afternoon; it's sort of an alternative to afternoon tea or a walk. I run through a series of about five or six exercises where I aim to hit different muscle groups. I start off with a stretch and five minutes of warm-up and go right into the lifts—usually performing three sets of eight to twelve repetitions each—and cool down with some more stretches and exercises for the core. The whole thing takes about an hour, give or take, and then I move on with my day.

My advice when you're beginning to build a fitness routine for yourself is to think about it as a plate filled with different kinds of food—main dishes, side dishes, meat, starch, and vegetables. My "main dish" in the gym is strength training—resistance-based exercises that create an athletic structure and enable me to do more physically. My side dishes are forms of exercise that target stretching, stability, and flexibility—all important for range of motion as well as mental preparation—and cardio-based activity like walking or jogging, which helps burn fat and strengthens the heart and lungs. To extend the analogy, it's up to you how you put together your meal—but you do need to include that crucial ingredient, strength training.

It's also up to you whether you prefer to work out around others at the gym or in the privacy of your own home. Both have advantages. By having some equipment at home, you can get right to work, saving time. On the other hand, there might be room to spread out and more and better equipment at a commercial gym. Just being around others tends to be motivating. If you do prefer to work out at home, you'll need some basic equipment such as resistance bands and maybe a kettlebell (more on this below). And of course, most important, you need to have the will to make it happen, not just once or twice, but consistently over weeks, months, and years. Here are some tips to get you started:

Start small and build up over time. The whole point of this is to build something that you can truly *own* and that lasts for the long term of your *life*. It's easy to start hard, overreach, and then get exhausted and quit. I've been there. Gyms have made an entire business model out of those New Year's memberships. It's so much better to start small, then build the practice and make it last. And for god's sake listen to your body: If a strength training exercise causes pain, stop the exercise; consider trying a lower weight or having a go at it again in a few days.

Understand that it takes time to see results, and enjoy where you are now. Women have been drilled to think of exercise as a way to do penance, to "work off" foods we later regret. The "I'll just walk it or run it off" mentality propagates a vicious cycle: a flurry of activity, then disappointment when it doesn't "work." Nothing is instant about this process. Strength training is a gradual build. Rather than thinking ahead to what you want to look or feel like in the future, enjoy being present in the moment, and savor the respite from your day that exercise provides. Working out is not punishment. Exercise and food have a symbiotic relationship, one that, when harnessed and maximized, can dramatically improve your physical health.

Save your cardio for the end of the workout. A lot of people think of cardio as a warm-up done at the beginning of the workout, but I disagree. If I do any cardio at all, it is at the end of the workout, because I don't want to steal any energy from my weightlifting output. For me, cardio is a release, and I make a point of bringing some aspect of cardio workouts outside if I can, even if it's cold or there's a light rain. I love walks and try to take one every day. Sometimes, if I know I need to miss the gym that day, I'll strap Velcro weights on my ankles and wrists to increase resistance and difficulty. Bikes, whether on the road or the stationary kind, can also be a terrific complement to strength training.

Don't feel like you have to do strength training every day. The good news is that you don't need to spend hours a day lifting weights to benefit from strength training. Significant improvement in strength often occurs with a few twenty- or thirty-minute weight-training sessions a week. To give the muscles time to recover, it's a good idea to rest one full day between exercising each specific muscle group. But repetition, creating a habit, is important.

I used to hate stretching. It felt like a waste of time. But now I see it as a way to limber up and get in the right head space before a workout begins. Stretching feels *nice*. And it does a lot for creating a positive mental space that signals "Ahhh, me time" before I get into my lifts.

Let's Start: Stretches

Stretching is the thing that I look forward to the most. I tweaked my mindset from thinking about stretching as injury prevention (the research is pretty mixed on that anyway) to more about creating a mindset to get into my body. Stretching is a treat, a moment to start activating your body. Stretching is really a bridge to strength training. So here I will take you through a typical stretch routine. There are so many ways to do it that you should really just do what feels good. My stretching sequence usually takes me 8 to 10 minutes.

Forward fold: Feet planted on the ground, lift your torso up, then fold forward and reach as far as you can. If I'm feeling particularly stiff, I like to pedal my knees a bit; after a few seconds I can feel my stretch deepen a little more. Then I reach farther down, maybe to my ankles. Eventually I can touch the floor. There's something about that that feels really good—like you can already see a benefit from giving yourself the time.

Side body bend: I then stretch my arms overhead. I use one hand to gently tug the other wrist toward that side of the body, then hold the stretch. Switch hands and do the same on the other side. This stretches out the side body of the upper torso. I also like to throw in some neck rolls here.

Downward dog to pigeon pose: Downward dog provides a nice stretch in the calves, which I pedal on either side before settling into a pigeon pose, where I bring one leg in front, knee bent, ankle on the floor, with the opposite leg behind, top of the foot planted down. If I'm feeling up to it, I'll fold my upper body forward or try to bend my upper body backward for a little stretch. See what you can do!

Then I do a little upper-body routine, which involves a **triceps stretch,** in which I lift one arm up and reach my hand behind my back to touch between my shoulder blades. I use the other hand to push the elbow above my shoulder back until I feel a nice stretch. Then I switch sides. After that, I do a **shoulder stretch,** crossing one arm across my chest and hugging it with the other arm at the elbow. Then switch.

Then, at the very end, I like to do a more active stretch—movements still in the spirit of stretching, but livelier—which starts to get the blood flowing and heart rate up a little more.

I'll start this portion with a bit of heel-toe walking, which helps warm up muscles around the shins and calves. I step one foot forward, planting the heel down and keeping the ankle flexed. I try to graze my fingertips or knuckles on the floor by bending over and feeling a stretch. Then I switch sides.

Next I'll go for a lunge and reach. Step forward, back knee bent, and reach. Sometimes I'll reach upward to the sky, then twist to the side for a more lateral stretch. On other days I like to anchor one arm to the ground and twist upward to the sky. I hold the pose for a few seconds and then switch sides.

Upper body swings: I have an old PVC pipe lying around the basement that I grab to stretch the upper body, sides, and shoulders. I like to grab one end of the pipe with each hand and move it around—first front to back, then side to side. If

I'm at the gym, I just swing my arms. It helps warm and loosen up muscles and joints.

My Top Ten Body-Weight Strength Movements

Now that you've finished with stretches, it's time to familiarize yourself with a series of exercises that rely on body weight to build strength. When people think of strength training, they usually think of all the gym equipment required, but in fact, many strength exercises can be done with little to no equipment. If you've got a body, you've got a gym. Sometimes to challenge myself, I try doing as many body-weight exercises as I can at home, without any additional equipment. Here are some of my greatest hits. You can do a couple of rounds, or circuits, of each of these. (One round of each of the exercises performed in a particular sequence is a circuit; if you go back and do another series of the same exercises, that's a second round or circuit, and so forth.)

While we're at it: A rep, or repetition, is a single execution of a particular exercise. (One chin-up? That's one rep. Ten chin-ups? That's ten reps.) A set refers to the exercise itself performed as a collection of reps. So three sets of ten push-ups looks like this: ten push-ups, followed by a minute or two of rest. Then another set of ten push-ups, followed by another break. Then the last ten push-ups. There, you've done three sets of ten reps each.

1. **Push-ups.** These make me feel like a badass G.I. Jane. Push-ups are the king (or should I say queen?) of all body-weight exercises, in my opinion, because they can be done anywhere

and in one simple movement do so much for so many different parts of the body. In general, push exercises tend to work the chest, but push-ups are a marvel in that they work not only chest muscles but also shoulders, abdominals, and even the upper back as well. Don't be shy starting with the assisted version, which is done with the knees down, and then working up to the unassisted version in an old-fashioned plank position. Each week I play with a few variations that work different muscle areas. For instance, you can position your hands wide apart or close together and point your hands inward or outward to hit different areas of the chest or focus more on the shoulders or triceps.

2. **Pull-ups.** If I'm not at a gym, I do pull-ups on a heavy iron clothesline rack anchored in my backyard. At my best, I can do ten in a row. After I got COVID, though, I needed help in getting back to finishing just one. If you are just starting out and have set yourself the goal of making it to one pull-up, try strapping bands to the post and placing your knees inside them, where they benefit from a little bounce and some support on the way up. These are great for developing lateral muscles in the back.

3. **Rows.** I like this exercise to work the back. You don't need a big rowing machine; these can be done with or without dumbbells, and they allow you to work one side at a time (With machines, sometimes you risk nudging your stronger side to work harder!) Resting one knee and one hand on a

bench (or chair or side of the bed), make a fist with the other hand and row upward. For more of a challenge, grab a soup can or a dumbbell in one hand. Be sure to keep the upper body upright in a neutral position. Switch sides to work the other arm.

4. **Squats.** I always feel like my butt could conquer the world after I do squats! Place your feet shoulder width or a little more apart, bend your knees, and thrust your hips/quads back like you're sitting in a chair. For added oomph, hold a weight in front of your chest or one in each hand. Dumbbells are great, but you can also use a filled milk jug or soup cans in each hand. Squats work the glutes, quadriceps, hamstrings, and calves.

5. **Lunges.** Besides helping build the glutes, quads, and hamstrings, lunges force you to work on stability—aka balance—a bit, thus engaging the core as well. Step forward, bending the forward knee to lower your body toward the ground, then walk the other leg forward. I like to stay low instead of popping back up; this makes the exercise more difficult. You can use dumbbells or soup cans in each hand for added weight and intensity.

6. **Planks.** I always marvel at how holding still can be so hard. I do planks at the very end of my workout as a wind-down. Planks engage not just the core muscles but the shoulders and arms as well.

7. **Donkey kicks.** I like to do these with a resistance band around my thighs (I keep these bands in a basket near the television) or at the end of a workout. Kneeling on all fours, kick one foot up toward the ceiling, keeping the knee bent. Do as many reps as possible; then switch to the other leg. These mostly target the glutes, but they also work the hamstrings, shoulders, and back a bit.

8. **Frog pumps.** Lie on your back on the floor. Bring the soles of your feet together, forming a diamond shape. Then lift your butt/hips off the ground for a count before setting them back down. That's one pump. Do as many reps as possible, focusing on squeezing the glutes. For added resistance, add a resistance band around your thighs. These activate the core, the glutes, and your hard-to-reach abductor muscles (those in the inner thighs).

9. **Monster walks.** I sometimes do these in the driveway. Put a resistance band around your thighs. In a half-squat position, keeping your glutes pushed back and your knees pressed out, walk ten paces forward, then ten paces backward. You can also do this walking side to side. For an extra challenge, add a band to the ankles as well. This is spectacular for adding strength and stability in the gluteus medius, which is the middle muscle in the butt.

10. **Dead bugs.** These are an incredibly effective abdominal exercise. I often wrap up a workout with dead bugs. Lying on my back with my lower back pressed to the ground, I slowly

bicycle my legs, one at a time, while keeping my arms stretched up to the ceiling. Sometimes I'll hold a weight in my hands while moving my legs, which makes it a little bit harder and adds resistance.

Perform a circuit by choosing five of these exercises, deciding ahead of time how many repetitions of the exercise you will aim for (six? eight? ten?) and how many rounds (two? three?). Each week, aim for another round, eventually getting to four circuits. Two to three times a week, add three abdominal exercises such as sit-ups, planks, and Russian twists (a sit-up variation in which you twist from side to side, elbow to knee). These basic, no-equipment exercises will offer you a solid foundation on which to build your practice.

When gyms closed during the pandemic and I had no equipment, I did a lot of these body-weight moves and found that they pushed my muscles in new ways and were easy to break up into different circuits.

Building Your Home Setup

If, after a couple of weeks of performing the body-weight exercises above, you want to deepen the work, you can add some toys and accessories. This is the equipment I think is most effective and valuable for building your personal gym.

Resistance Bands

I highly recommend you start by purchasing some inexpensive lightweight resistance bands, which are great for targeting hard-to-reach areas and working specific small muscle groups such as those in the inner thighs or abdomen. A 2019 Brazilian study that compared the impact on muscular strength of resistance bands as opposed to conventional devices (dumbbells, machines) showed that the bands promoted similar strength gains to conventional devices.[1] And a 2022 study revealed that resistance band training lowered body fat in overweight people better than other forms of training, including free weights.[2]

Resistance bands can be used on their own for upper-body exercises: One way I exercise my lats, for instance, is by grabbing the ends of the bands with both hands and pulling the band out horizontally. But I also like to use them to deepen the difficulty of certain lower body exercises such as squats or donkey kicks.

Another big benefit of resistance bands is their portability. While dumbbells and and other types of weights can be clunky and take up a lot of room, resistance bands occupy virtually no space at all and can cost as little as a few dollars. I always pack some into my luggage and in the trunk of my car whenever I travel.

On a trip near a beach or a pretty trail, I've tied a couple of bands to a post or a tree and used them as resistance for squats and, using the same setup, as an alternative to cable pull-throughs or cable kick-backs, which are excellent for glute muscles.

Kettlebells

These are perfect if you're ready to keep building your arsenal. Kettlebells can be used to increase the load in certain exercises and challenge the muscles. A single twelve-kilogram (twenty-six-pound) kettlebell has been a good weight for me, personally. You can also buy adjustable ones that can be dialed up or down in weight (though I've always found these clunky and unwieldy).

I often start my workout with some kettlebell swings as a warmup. A study published in *The Journal of Strength and Conditioning Research* demonstrates[3] that the mechanical demands of the swing exercise are comparable with—and in some cases exceed—the demands of other forms of resistance exercises.

I find that swings with the kettlebell are a great full-body activator, and I love that I can feel different muscle groups working, particularly those in the posterior chain—the ones in the back—such as my hamstrings, glutes, and back muscles. The swinging motion is kind of enjoyable, and I love that it gives me a core workout, too.

Barbells and Dumbbells

These weights are the classic strength-training tools. While the big clunky machines that you see at the gym are fine for targeting and isolating certain muscle groups and they're quick to use, as they're already set up for what they're supposed to do, barbells and dumbbells actually end up working more muscle groups because they recruit helper muscles, such as those in the core, for stabilizing. And they're easy to keep at home.

When looking to set up my home gym during the pandemic, I saved money by buying used equipment. After all, weights don't wear out! I have an Olympic barbell, the seven-foot-long, forty-five-pound solid steel center of my workout life. I have cast-iron pairs of plates for the barbell ranging from two and a half pounds to forty-five pounds. My dumbbells are a mix of steel ones and those coated with rubber. A squat rack and bench complete my setup.

Bench

An exercise bench is basically a padded board that you can set at different angles, allowing you to multiply the types of lifts you are able to do: lifting weights while lying flat on the bench or at an incline or seated upright. It's narrow enough that it can be stowed away pretty easily.

Optional Extras

Suspension-training straps. These straps can be mounted at home from the ceiling or on the back of a door. They allow you to utilize both gravity and body weight through various push and pull exercises. Such a strap is a very useful tool and takes up hardly any room. TRX is the commonly used brand, but there are cheaper knock-offs available.

Velcro weights. I keep a basket of these by the front door, when I feel like giving my regular dog walk a little extra juice. I strap one on each ankle and wrist, and this makes my muscles work a little bit harder on a routine walk, particularly uphill. Be careful taking them off when you get home. It can take a woozy minute or two to get used to the shift in weight, as everything will feel much lighter!

Hip bands. These are different from the long resistance bands I describe above. They're shorter, meant to fit snugly around your thighs. I wear them to help accentuate work on the rear in exercises that target the glutes such as squats, donkey kicks, frog pumps, and the like.

Yoga ball. I have a big inflatable ball that I used during pregnancy, and I've just kept it. I like to use it for ab work (for different styles of crunches) but also sometimes instead of the workout bench. The bit of instability produced by the ball makes the core work a little harder.

My Favorite Weighted Strength Exercises

Here are some of the workouts I do with my home gym setup. These can be adjusted for any level of fitness. It's very important to use proper technique when training with weights to avoid injuries. Those new to weight training can go to my Instagram @AnneMarieChaker to work out with me. You can also work out with a trainer, at least to start.

My favorite approach is to divvy up workouts across the week, focusing on only certain related muscle groups at a time. This encourages a systematic approach, and I enjoy feeling the progression of having worked my full body through the course of the seven days. A classic way might be to start with a leg day (focused on the quadriceps, the muscles at the front of the leg); then moving to the back and biceps, which are connected and work together; before bringing in the chest and triceps, which are also connected and complementary; and adding a second leg day (focused on the back muscles, hamstrings, and glutes). The other benefit to working muscle groups together is that you can give them a proper rest—ideally forty-eight hours—before putting them to work again, which helps them heal and grow stronger.

Day 1: Legs

Legs anchor the weight of the body, but in the weight room, they often don't get enough love. While for many people the focus is on the upper body, the lower body requires more work, because it includes larger muscle groups that use more energy from the heart and the brain. So the first leg day of the week is sort of my "big macro" leg day, where I hit the big compound movements (which, while leg focused, work multiple muscle groups across the body).

Squat

The squat is a great compound lift that works the big muscles like the quads and glutes but also forces you to work on balance and stability. And when you do that, you are working muscles all over the body, from those in the core to the calves.

In the basic barbell squat, the bar itself is forty-five pounds, so that may well be enough for many people to get started. Hoist the bar from the rack onto your upper back, below the shoulders. With hips back, knees shoulder width apart, and toes pointed slightly out, initiate the squat by bending the knees until your butt is parallel to the ground. Keeping the core braced and the chest up, rise back up until you are upright to complete one repetition.

With squats, multiple muscle groups are engaged—the glutes, quadriceps, hamstrings, and calves as well as muscles in the core and the lower back. It's about as full body a workout as you can get from one single exercise.

There are also a host of variations to mix in on different days:

- **Goblet Squat:** Squat exercises performed holding a dumbbell against the chest under the chin.

- **Sissy Squat:** Squats performed with a band looped around a post, feet placed inside with the band strapped around the thighs to provide support and resistance.

- **Bulgarian Split Squat:** Single-legged squats performed with one foot resting on a bench.

Deadlift

Deadlifts are big compound movements that work the entire body. The process of anchoring, pressing down to the floor, and lifting heavy weight with correct form is something that makes me feel like the strongest of athletes. This particular lift tends to focus on the posterior chain, or the muscles on the back of the body.

Place a loaded barbell on the ground. Standing a couple of inches in front of it, feet shoulder width apart, grab the barbell (hands placed just outside the legs). Using your lower body, pressing your feet into the floor, lift the barbell until you are standing upright and holding it. Drop the barbell. That's one repetition. As with squats, deadlifts are also considered a compound exercise that works multiple major muscle groups: the glutes, hamstrings, core, and back. Different placements of the hands on the bar and of the feet can help shift the focus to different muscle groups that you want to work. My two favorites:

- **Sumo Deadlift:** Place your feet wide apart, with your toes pointed out. Your hands are placed closer together (inside the width of the legs). This hand and foot placement really ensures a focus on the glute muscles. On the lift I like to think of pushing the ground away with my feet, to really engage the muscles.

- **Romanian Deadlift:** This is similar to a conventional deadlift but targets the glutes and hamstrings a little more. Your feet are placed a little closer together—about eight inches to a foot apart—with the bar placed just below the knees, which are not too bent. The lift is performed by pushing the feet into the ground to lift the bar—engaging the glutes, hamstrings, and core—before bringing it back down, not necessarily touching the floor but just below the knees.

Leg Press

Most people don't have a leg press at home, so using this device is something generally done at the gym. It works the front of the quads. I like to take advantage of the leg press on the days when I'm at the gym.

Load the plates before sitting down, and press without locking the knees completely. I like to do pyramids, where I keep loading on forty-five-pound plates (or whatever size you like) for a goal of six to eight repetitions per set until it's really hard to push even one rep; then I take one off progressively, set by set. Like the deadlift and the squat, the leg press helps develop lower body muscles. The main difference is it is performed on a machine, which means it does a better job of isolating the quads, glutes, hamstrings, and calves without getting the core and the back involved as much.

Lunges

Take advantage of a backyard, a driveway, or a length of space in a gym that nobody's using.

Step forward until your front leg is at a ninety-degree angle. Trying not to come all the way up, move your back leg forward and repeat. Staying low adds difficulty to the lunges. You can also hold weights in each hand for added intensity, developing the glutes, quads, hamstrings, and calves.

At the gym, leg curl and leg extension machines are usually set side by side, and I like to do them in tandem because they are complementary: Curls work the back of the leg, extensions the front.

Leg Curls

Leg curls work the hamstrings and glutes. You can achieve this with the traditional leg curl machine at the gym, by lying down on your stomach and curling your weighted feet upward toward your butt. If you're at home—or even at the gym while someone else is using the leg curl machine—you can squeeze a dumbbell between your feet while lying down on a bench for a similar result.

Leg Extensions

While seated at the machine, lock your feet into weights and kick upward for more quad-focused work. When I'm staying in hotels, I've used Velcro ankle weights to do leg extensions. This method is surprisingly effective at high reps of twelve to fifteen per set!

Abductors/Adductors

Abductors work the outside portion of your glutes, while adductors work the inside of your thighs. There are machines at the gym to help you achieve this, but you can also use resistance bands to work these areas. For adductors, I place a band around my upper thighs and lie down on my side. Keeping my toes touching, I perform clamshells, opening and closing my knees while engaging the thighs. Then for abductors, I like to place a band around my upper thighs, and while seated with my feet on the floor, push outward for one rep. In both cases, you can aim for as many reps as possible, or AMRAP.

Day 2: Back/Shoulders

The back and shoulders are related muscle groups, so it's natural to do exercises that target them together. The muscles involved include lats, rhomboids, traps, and scapulae. You can also think of the exercises that hit these groups as more of the pull type.

Lat Pull-Downs

These work the lats and biceps and are performed seated in front of the pull-down bar (if you're at the gym). Leaning back ever so slightly, hold the bar with a wide grip (outside the armpits), pull it down to chest height, and allow it to return to the starting position, while keeping some tension, for one rep. You can also perform these with over-the-door straps or bands at home.

Straight-Arm Pull-Downs

This variation of the lat pull-down works the triceps and upper back muscles a little more. Standing in front of the pull-down bar (I like to use a shorter bar for this exercise), which has been set high above your head, pull the bar all the way down for one repetition, and slowly return the bar back up, holding some tension. This can also be done at home with a long-enough resistance band tied to a high-enough post.

Seated Cable Rows

At a cable machine, sit with your feet planted in front of you, maintaining a slight bend in the knees. While keeping the upper body stable, pull the V-bar to your chest. Then keeping your hands on the bar and holding some tension, return the bar gently to the starting position. This can also be performed at home, in a pinch. While seated, loop a resistance band around the bottom of your feet. Gripping one end of the band with each hand, perform rows.

Dumbbell Rows

This version allows focus on training one side at a time, which I like because I feel my right side tends to be slightly stronger. Place one knee and the hand from the same side of the body in front of you on a bench. With the opposite hand, hold the dumbbell near your calf and pull it up to your armpit level for one repetition.

Complete a number of reps on one side before switching to the other.

Pull-Ups

There's nothing more rewarding than being able to increase your reps of these over time, and seeing yourself progress is very fun. Holding an overhead bar so that your feet are dangling off the ground, pull yourself up until your chin is over the bar. For an assist, you can loop a resistance band to the bar and place one knee inside it. When I'm at home, I have an outdoor steel clothesline bar that happens to double as a handy pull-up bar. Many people purchase doorframe pull-up bar kits to install their own home version indoors.

Back Extension

I like this one because it gives me a glute workout as well. Anchoring your feet down on an incline bench, hinge at the hips and lift up without rounding your back; then return to the starting position. For added difficulty, you can hold a plate at your chest while doing this exercise.

Reverse Fly

This exercise is for the muscles in the upper back and shoulders. Standing with your feet shoulder width apart and your knees slightly bent, hinge your hips back and angle your chest forward. Holding a dumbbell in each hand, with a slight bend in the elbows, open your arms wide to the sides while inhaling, then down on the exhale.

Day 3: Chest/Triceps

Some women wonder why they should bother working their chest muscles. But since every part of the body is connected, working the front of the upper body helps build symmetry as well as strengthen muscles in your core and the backs of your arms. Chest muscles are important for supporting your breasts by way of the muscles underneath the breast tissue.

Chest exercises are typically push exercises. Think about what's engaged when you push a sled or do a push-up: The triceps are often also in play. Triceps make up about two-thirds of the arm, so toning them up will also help strengthen the arm.

Bench Press

This is the exercise I always start a chest day with. The bench press is a compound exercise that works multiple muscle groups in the upper body, including the pectoral muscles, the arms, the shoulders, and the core. Most people like to start their workouts with the compound exercises because they use the most energy. Tiring out the triceps before hitting the bench press won't give you the best results on the bench. Do the big exercises that take the most energy first.

Lying faceup on a bench, holding either a barbell or a pair of dumbbells, one in each hand, press the weight up until your arms are straight, then bring it back down to chest level. If you are using a barbell, make sure there is a rack behind you to anchor the weight on after you're done, and ask for someone to spot you, ready to grab the barbell if you need a boost.

Dips

I like to do these in between bench press sets because they can be done easily with the bench. Sit on the edge of the bench with your hands behind you, palms down on the bench. Stick your legs straight out in front of you, heels down and toes pointed upward. (For a less intense version, bend your knees and put your feet flat on the floor.) Elbows bent, drop your butt off the bench and dip it down until it is near the floor, keeping your butt close to the bench behind you. You should feel the work in your triceps. Then push back up to your original position for one rep.

Incline Dumbbell Press

This variation of the dumbbell press starts with the bench set at an incline. It works the upper portion of the chest and the shoulders more. I also like that it works each side more individually. Holding dumbbells in each hand, push them up overhead until your arms are locked straight up. Then bring the dumbbells down until they are nearly touching the front of your chest, right by your shoulders, and your arms are bent at a 90-degree angle.

Cable Crossovers

These are a good alternative to bench presses that help activate the chest muscles in a different way. The use of cables provides a novel angle and type of resistance, where I also feel resistance on the release, which forces my body to adjust and new muscles to be activated. The name of the game in strength training is to hit muscles from all angles and in different ways to produce a rich result.

Standing with your back toward the cable machine, place your feet in a staggered stance, one in front of the other. Grab the handles of the machine and drive your hands forward, allowing them to pass with one hand above and one below in front of your belly. Return to the starting position and repeat, alternating the hand that goes on top.

Dumbbell Fly

Lie on your back on the bench, a dumbbell in each hand. Open your arms wide, then press the weights up and bear hug them together while keeping an imaginary ball in between you and your arms. Then open out the arms back wide. I like that dumbbell flies are a strengthener but also open the chest and increase range of motion, which helps reduce tightness and pain and feels good.

Push-Ups

As mentioned above, push-ups are the go-anywhere chest exercise. To make push-ups easier, do them with your knees on the floor. Another assisted version involves placing your hands up on a bench, which works the shoulders more.

Day 4: Second Leg Day (Glute-Focused) and Biceps

This is a second leg day, and on this day, I might focus more on the glutes, pulling from exercises I didn't do on the first leg day and adding in a couple of variations.

On this day, I'll throw in a variation on squats that focuses on the glutes a bit more. One week I might pick one of the following:

Goblet Squats

This exercise is great because it can be done anywhere; you don't have to have a big squat-rack setup. Plant your feet slightly wider than shoulder width, toes pointed out. Hold a dumbbell (or a heavy jug or any other substitute weight) in front of your chest under your chin. Push your hips back and squat until your butt is parallel to the ground. Then drive back up.

Banded Sissy Squats

Wrap a three-foot band to a post, step inside the band, and lean back slightly while squatting. The pressure from the band intensifies and assists the squatting motion.

Hack Squats

These are done on a hack-squat machine at the gym. Placing plates for weight, position your feet shoulder width apart and release the safety handle. Squat until your legs are at a 90-degree angle, then drive back up.

Sumo Deadlift

Place your feet wide apart (beyond shoulder width), with toes pointed out. Grab a weighted barbell and raise it (and yourself) to standing. I like to think of pressing my feet down and apart while I do this to activate the glutes.

Hip Thrusts

These are a pain in the neck to set up, but worth it in that I think they are one of the best exercises for glute building.

Lean a bench against a wall and lie faceup on it. The bench should hit just below your shoulder blades, and your feet should be about shoulder width apart. Place padding on your lap (I use a cushion or a rolled-up yoga mat) before hoisting a barbell on top of it. With the weighted barbell balanced at the hips, lower your butt down to the floor, then bring it back up by pushing your hips up parallel to the floor. You can also find machines now at the gym for performing this exercise, but having the barbell in play, I think, forces some stability work and therefore activates the core, which is a nice plus.

Cable Kickbacks

Cables are a great way to mix in a different type of resistance than standard weights; cables force the body to work at different angles and challenge stability, which works different muscle groups. At a gym's cable machine, adjust the setting so the ankle-strap attachment is anchored near the floor. Wrap the ankle strap around one ankle. Feet together, lean forward slightly and kick that leg up and back. Repeat with the other leg. If you don't have access to a cable machine, you can also perform kickbacks while holding on to the back of a chair for support. Sometimes I wrap on ankle weights I have lying around the house to do these, or tie a resistance band around a post to do smaller kickbacks, or pulses.

Bicep Curls

Hold a dumbbell in each hand. Curl one dumbbell close to the shoulder; then curl the other. (This can also be done with a barbell using both hands at once.)

Chin-Up

While a pull-up uses a pronated grip, with the palms facing away, the palms in a chin-up face toward the body, a supinated grip, to target the biceps a little more.

What to Do When You Just Don't Feel Like It

Sometimes we just don't feel like getting up and working out. It's hard to move out of our comfort zone. We are conditioned to want to feel comfortable, not uncomfortable. Being a badass athlete isn't about what you can do on a specific day. It's really about having the discipline to get off your butt and move each and every day. And just getting started is 90 percent of the battle.

Here are a few of my hacks that often help me get over the hump on those days when I just don't feel like it.

Motivational Hack 1: Try coffee and Motown. A little caffeine really does help. According to the International Society of Sports Nutrition, caffeine in the amounts of .9 to 2.7 mg per pound of body weight is actually helpful to workout performance.[4] There are so many pre-workout beverages on the market, and most of them contain caffeine. I like to pour myself half a cup of coffee and put on some music—in my case Motown (musical Prozac!), but you should go with whatever elevates your mood or that you know will help you get moving.

Motivational Hack 2: Treat yourself. Give yourself a little something special for your workout, either afterward or before. If I'm in a health club that has one, I especially love a dip in the cold plunge afterward. It is so refreshing and invigorating and offers a little bit of a mood boost. Or in the winter, I might spend some time in the sauna. If I work out at home, I might follow the workout with a bath filled with Epsom salts, which help with muscle soreness. Or it could be simply listening to new music or wearing a new T-shirt or sports bra. Anything that makes you feel a little bit excited or puts a pep in your step.

Motivational Hack 3: Start easy. Really, just move. And one way to ease your body in is by starting with some stretching. For me, stretching is a way to feel good and get moving. It's sort of a little treat to your body and a bridge from not moving to moving. It doesn't have to be super involved; I like to aim for five decent stretches, and sometimes they naturally flow one into the other, depending on how I'm feeling.

I think the best piece of advice I can give you as you begin your strength-training practice is to avoid wanting to see differences in your body right away. These things take time. Instead, focus on the pleasure of the routine. When I step into the gym, there is a rubbery smell of equipment. I associate that smell with me time, so even before I do a single exercise, I already feel better. This investment of time and energy belongs to you—it's a space you've carved out from the bustle of life to take care of yourself. Put the emphasis on the feelings of accomplishment you get throughout your workout: the pleasure you gain from moving, the sensation of your muscles being activated, and after you've completed an exercise, the satisfaction of finishing.

When I interviewed Maria Colacurcio, a forty-eight-year-old founder and chief executive of a pay-equity software company, it became clear that her motivation came from a deeper place than wanting to see differences in her body. Maria balances her career with mothering seven children ages three to seventeen and an intense competition and training schedule. She competes in Hyrox races: 1-kilometer runs interspersed with eight high-intensity workout stations.

To prepare for the three to four of these races she does each year, she trains six times a week for about an hour, usually while it's still dark and before her kids wake up, in the solace of her garage gym. Sometimes if she can't finish a workout, she splits it in two, doing the strength training in the morning and a forty-minute running exercise after the workday is done.

Knowing she is going to compete against other athletes who also train hard is something she relishes and looks forward to. She loves having a goal in sight. But most of all, she sees her training as cherished moments devoted to herself. And having that makes her disciplined about everything else she has going on in her life.

"I feel it especially when I'm doing a pull-up," she says. "There's something about being able to do that that embeds into every other part of my life. I literally pull myself up. There's something about that connection—whether professionally or being more of a positive, engaged parent—about being able to lift yourself up, lift heavy things."

Very little of what drives Maria, however, is about trying to see changes in her physique. Her approach to food is about eating to fuel performance. "I've gained pounds," she says, but her body composition is leaner and more muscular. When she found strength training, she says, "I had to eat to be strong, and with Hyrox, if you don't fuel, you can't perform."

The biggest reason people quit is they want the gratification of seeing changes in their bodies right away. But the real power of this practice is not what's happened to your body. That's the gravy. The power is in the attention you are paying to yourself and your growth. It's also in the focus on strength, doing something hard when life pulls you in many different directions. So take pleasure in taking care of yourself. When you enter the gym or the basement or even just plop down a mat in the corner of your bedroom, appreciate what you're about to do. I like to have a little mantra, something I say to myself to get in the right mood, while I'm stretching, in the sauna, or during my initial warm-up: "This is my time, for me, to build myself up."

The Importance of Rest Days

I make sure to take two to three rest days a week. Rest days are just as crucial as training days, important not only to prevent burnout but also to allow time for your muscles to grow. You can't make gains in your health and physique if you are not taking time for recovery. When you give your muscles a rest, you can more easily tackle the exercises in the next workout, becoming a better athlete who can handle progressively more pressure. Learning the value and importance of rest—physiological and mental—is just as vital as knowing how to train.

When we work out, we are intentionally breaking down our body and fatiguing our muscles. This muscle damage initiates a process in which certain hormones, along with protein, synthesize new cells used to repair the damaged muscle fibers.

Rest is what allows for that process to work. Muscles don't grow during training—they grow during recovery. After a workout, your muscles build new protein in a process called protein synthesis, which in turn stimulates their growth. The elevation in protein synthesis happens very quickly after a training session, with most research showing it to peak anywhere in the five- to twenty-four-hour period after a training session. This means that muscles start the process of growth within hours after a session, and this process continues at least for the next day, if not longer.

In a 1995 study published in the *Canadian Journal of Applied Physiology*, where subjects did twelve sets of bicep curls, researchers found that the subjects' protein synthesis was elevated by 50 percent at four hours following training, peaking at 109 percent at twenty-four hours before slowing considerably by thirty-six hours.[5] And so an ideal training frequency would therefore allow for a rest period of twenty-four to forty-eight hours, giving the muscle groups time to grow and reap the maximum benefits of protein synthesis before they are trained again.

Some people tend to want to work out seemingly nonstop. It can sometimes get a little addictive, and I've been there. But that is actually counterproductive—causing strain, fatigue, burnout, and susceptibility to injury. You should aim for no more than four workouts a week to start, mixing up the muscle groups you're working on and taking at least three full days of rest interspersed between the workout days. And listen to your body: You'll know if you feel like you're overdoing it. If three days in a row feels like too much, do two days in a row. Take rest days back to back if you feel you need to. Start gradually rather than taking on too much too soon and then feeling overwhelmed or disappointed (or injuring yourself).

A 2011 study examined how sleep deprivation affects muscle gain by following individuals who were on a strict sleep schedule for 72 hours.[6] During this time, one group was allowed 5.5 hours of sleep per day, the other 8.5 hours. All individuals followed a calorie-regulated diet. Researchers found that those who slept only 5.5 hours had 60 percent less muscle mass by the end of the study, while those who slept 8.5 hours had 40 percent more.

Besides improving musculature and physical development, sleep also helps to improve the quality of workouts. A 2015 study published in *Physiology & Behavior* measured the quality of the serves of college tennis players when they increased their sleep to at least nine hours each day.[7] Serves improved to 42 percent accuracy from 35 percent. In another study, numerous improvements were found among Stanford University basketball players after periods of sleeping ten hours a night: Their sprints were faster, their free-throw percentages increased by at least 9 percent, and they reported a better overall sense of well-being.[8]

If you're feeling the need to do something a little bit active on a rest day, here are a few ideas.

Stretching: Stretching is typically performed before or after a workout, to loosen up or cool down. But I also like to do stretches on my off days. I really take the time, since my body has a tendency to feel tight, which can inhibit range of motion in my lifting. I also like how it helps me decompress and clears my mind. My greatest hits include an upper body stretch (arms to the sky, stretch, and then lightly tug on one arm, then the other); a seated forward bend (seated, feet stretched out in front, holding nose to knees as far as possible and hands to feet); knees to chest (back on the floor, cycling one knee to chest, hold, then the other); and downward dog (heels up, heels down) followed by child's pose. This quick routine takes all of eight to ten minutes, but it feels as refreshing and therapeutic as a nap. On good-weather days, I take a mat or a blanket and do this outside. On cold days, I like to go cozy and light a candle at home, to really bring on the tranquility.

Restorative yoga: This type of yoga prioritizes relaxing, regrouping, holding gentle poses, and staying still. Numerous studies have shown that restorative yoga helps slow breathing, reduces blood pressure, and produces a sense of calm and well-being. I recently started practicing once a week on an off day. It can be incredibly challenging to make myself be still, open up, and stretch. I pick three to five poses and use bolsters and blankets that I have around the house. My favorites include a supported version of legs up the wall, child's pose, spinal twists, and a seated bend over legs.

Meditation: I like to think of meditation as bodybuilding for the mind. It's a practice that trains your mind to be present in the moment and has been shown to help improve focus and concentration. Research also indicates that meditation can decrease symptoms of depression and anxiety and induce lasting positive changes in the brain.[9] It took me a while to get into meditation, but now I do it for about fifteen to twenty minutes once or twice a week, using guidance from either the Peloton app or YouTube. As author and psychologist Daniel Goleman says in a 2017 column, edited by my *Wall Street Journal* colleague Elizabeth Bernstein:

> *There are many beneficial effects of this simple exercise. Attention strengthens. Concentration improves. Memory improves. Learning improves. And because the same circuitry in the brain that focuses your attention also manages the amygdala, which causes you to get anxious or upset or depressed, people have a double benefit: They react less strongly to things that used to upset them and recover more quickly when they do get upset.*[10]

Walking: When the weather is decent, I love going out for a stroll, not to sneak in a cardio workout, but just to move a bit and to feel the wind or sun on my face. Walking can also be a form of meditation. A no-agendas walk can be a mindful, focused practice, and a great way to bond with a friend or family member. I recommend it as an alternative to meeting for a drink.

Women tend to feel guilty about self-care. I know I did for a long time. I felt I was being selfish—*I should be spending this time parenting. I should be doing something with the kids. I should be helping them do their homework.* But showing your children how you choose to treat yourself, to respect yourself and care for yourself, is perhaps one of the greatest gifts you can give them—because chances are they will adopt the same behavior for themselves and model it for their own children.

CHAPTER 7

EAT LIKE A BODYBUILDER

The Value of Protein and Other Macronutrients

Before I became a bodybuilder, food used to be something I minimized, trying to eat as little as I could so that I could be thin, or binging and feeling bad afterward. The biggest shift since I've started training is that I eat more, and more consistently, making sure I'm getting the most bang out of my food and maximizing nutrients. My focus is on real, whole foods, minimizing my consumption of processed and ultra-processed foods as much as possible.

Too often in my life, food has ended up being a last-minute affair. If there wasn't anything in the fridge, I turned to something quick and ready-made. For years, I dealt with the question "What am I going to eat for dinner?" only when I was hungry. That meant the choices I made were often less than great—takeout, empty calories, and the inevitable overeating—because they were rushed and the result of necessity. What I've discovered is that when I plan ahead and prepare food from scratch, nourishing myself is no longer an afterthought. I'm able to let go of binging and restricting cycles. I usually set aside time on Sunday to do a big grocery shop and then chop and prepare vegetables and proteins. (I aim to do this again, on a smaller scale, some time midweek.) It doesn't have to look beautiful or fancy. But it's nutritious and whole, and that's what matters.

A friend of mine asked me how I eat, and when I started to explain that I spend some time each week prepping my food and stocking my fridge, he said, "But I just don't want to obsess about food that much." I thought about that. Here's the thing: You're going to obsess about it anyway. We all obsess about food. If we don't know what to eat, we skip a meal and either end up cranky or reach for easy foods with little sustenance. We're all eventually going to think about food and make a decision. So we might as well make it a healthful one.

In the past, I was easily drawn to all kinds of diet trends. I covered food trends for years for *The Wall Street Journal* and other publications. You name it and I've written about it: The ketogenic diet, plant-based "meats," collagen-infused foods, and certain ingredients that go viral—a sudden national obsession with a single ingredient like sweet potato or cauliflower and an attempt to turn it into everything from pizza crust to rice.

The main thing I've learned from my training as a bodybuilder is that none of these labels means anything and that we make nutrition way more complicated than it has to be. There are no good foods or bad foods. Foods are choices we make. That's it. Sometimes, if I'm training to compete or have a particular body goal in mind, my choices will reflect my physical goals. Sometimes I make choices for sheer pleasure. Depending on where I am in life, those choices are all okay, and I don't let food control me. I make my decisions and own them. I may decide to choose a beautiful restaurant meal with my loved ones or a slice of birthday cake or pizza with the family. But I own that choice and refuse to feel guilty about it.

Diets are all about restriction. The foods on any given diet are boring and unappealing, and people begin to feel stifled and irritable. Then they binge and fall off the wagon and end up gaining the weight right back. A 2013 review published in *Frontiers in Psychology* showed that fifteen out of twenty studies of dieting measures predicted that teens and adults following a diet would gain weight.[1]

But the way I like to think about food is from a place of positivity, not negativity: I am making decisions that optimize the way I want my body to look, prioritizing the foods it needs to function best. Rather than fixating on what I can't or shouldn't have, I think about what I am *choosing* to eat. This simple mindset shift—of putting a plus sign next to food rather than a minus—has completely altered my approach toward how I want to nourish myself.

Contrast this with the weeks before a competition, when I have to reduce calories in order to lean out and showcase the muscle I've built. Muscle normally is hidden by a healthy layer of fat, and when we prep for competition, we strip away the fat to show off the body we've worked on building in the off-season. That lean-and-mean version is how the public likes to think of a bikini body, but such a body is not one intended to function in real life. I try to remember that the reduction in calories is temporary, and in the weeks after a competition, I go back to eating well and plentifully in order to build up my body. That place is where my body operates the best.

The sport of bodybuilding is largely about maximizing nutrition for body goals based around the development of muscle and the control of fat, which we call sculpting a physique. The way bodybuilders think about food is in terms of three macronutrients: proteins, carbohydrates, and fats. Macronutrients, which I'll break down in this chapter, are the nutrients your body needs in large amounts, to provide the energy required for basic bodily functions, everything from breathing to walking. The reason bodybuilders think about macros rather than calories is that macronutrients can be more specifically measured when it comes to shaping the body. Protein is important for muscle building and an athletic physique. Most people eat around 10 to 20 percent protein, but it's actually best to get your protein closer to around a third of your diet. Carbohydrates are important for the long term. They also help us build our physiques and provide energy. And fats are important to help digest the other nutrients but should be used judiciously.

Here are my tips for understanding and embracing the three macronutrient groups.

Ditch the Fear of Carbs

Carbohydrates are our main source of energy; they provide the body with glucose, which is converted to energy used to support physical activity and processes like digestion. When you're trying to build an athletic frame, eating enough carbohydrates is essential, so that your body has energy to recover your muscles. Without enough energy stored in carbs, the body turns to proteins to keep you going, which can lead to muscle loss. While carbs get a bad rap in diet books and on food labels, about half of what we eat typically comes from carbohydrates. Carbs not only help us function but also provide satiety, making us feel full and satisfied.

Carbs are found in potatoes, rice, bread, cereals, and other grains, but it may surprise you to learn that fruits and vegetables are also made up mostly of carbs. If someone tells you that they are watching their carbs and then grabs a salad, know that they are grabbing ... carbs. Which, I think, underscores the silliness of treating carbs like the enemy, as you can see from the chart below:

Food	Carbohydrates (grams)
Tossed green salad (3 cups) without dressing	13
½ salt bagel	13
1 cup broccoli	6
200 g cooked white rice	56
200 g cooked brown rice	45
200 g cooked quinoa	39

Source: MyFitnessPal

About half, if not more, of our calories each day should come from carbs, so how did this category of food get such a bad reputation? The reason is partly because so many of the carbs in our food ecosystem are the processed, refined kind, like white rice, white bread, pasta, and breakfast cereal. When carbs are processed, many of their nutrients and most of their fiber gets removed. This means that when you eat these kinds of carbs, they can cause your blood sugar to spike. Once your blood sugar spikes and then crashes, you're going to want another hit of those carbs, which can lead to overeating. Blood sugar spikes are often associated with weight gain and, in some cases, diabetes. All of which is to say that it's fine to eat processed and refined carbs now and then, but it's better to aim for nutrient-dense sources of carbs, like brown rice, whole grain bread, oats, and other whole grains, as well as all fresh vegetables. They are more fibrous and rich in vitamins and other nutrients, and you will *feel* better consuming them.

Prioritize Protein

Protein is the most important macronutrient for building muscle. Organs, tissues, muscles, and hormones are all made from protein. When protein is digested, it's broken up into amino acids, which are the building blocks of tissues. Those amino acids help repair and maintain muscle tissue that gets torn up during a workout, thus helping us build more of it.

The number one thing to understand about protein is that most of us don't get enough of it, particularly women, who have been conditioned to order the salad or skip a meal in favor of green juice. If you eat a classic Western diet, you probably get about 50 percent of your energy from carbs, 35 percent from fats, and only 15 percent from protein.[2] Compare this to estimates of the preagricultural diet of our hunter-gatherer ancestors, who may have obtained as much as one-third of their energy from protein.[3] We're eating less protein now in part because there are so many other options in the yummy, snacky world of packaged foods in the modern diet.

The U.S. Food and Nutrition Board sets the Recommended Dietary Allowance (RDA) for protein at only 0.8 grams per kilogram of body weight each day. So for a 140-pound person, that's about 50 grams of protein per day (an omelet with cheese for breakfast) and for a 200-pound person, that's about 70 grams of protein (a full breakfast with multiple eggs, sausage, and bacon).

But critics say that calculation is a bare minimum. If you're exercising, you need to eat a lot more protein than that, especially if you're trying to build a strong body with muscle mass. As an article from Harvard Health Publishing points out, the RDA for protein is "the minimum amount you need to keep from getting sick—not the specific amount you are supposed to eat every day."[4]

Most young adults tend to consume close to the recommended amounts of protein. But as a study from 2019 found, later in life, about 30 percent of men in their fifties and sixties fall short, and nearly half of women aged fifty and older do. This is because, as we age, our bodies stop processing protein as efficiently, and we need to eat more of it to maintain our muscle mass and strength. We need protein for our cells—including muscle cells—and our bodies constantly recycle whatever protein we consume, providing us with the amino acids that become the building blocks of the new proteins our bodies need. The goal is to consume protein from food at a faster rate than our body is breaking it down. Eating enough protein helps retain muscle mass while resistance training.

For example, a woman in midlife looking to lift weights regularly and to build muscle mass would want to consume about a gram of protein per pound of ideal body weight each day, if not more. If you're 150 pounds, you should be looking at eating 150 grams of protein each day, which could look like: three eggs for breakfast, a chicken breast for lunch, and a piece of salmon for dinner, with a couple of protein-rich snacks like Greek yogurt and a scoop of protein powder in a drink along the way. I'm going to guess that you probably eat a lot less than this currently, but it's not too late to rethink how you eat.

A position paper published by the International Society of Sports Nutrition says that much higher amounts of protein (2.3 to 3.1 grams per kilogram per day) are needed to retain muscle mass in athletes who are cutting weight.[5] This higher level of protein intake may have positive effects on body composition, such as promoting fat loss, according to this same paper.

The good news about protein is that among other things, it helps you feel full. "There's definitely a relationship between protein and satiety, and their effect on hormones," says Barbara Davis, a registered dietitian and regulatory expert in Canton, Connecticut.[6] As she explains, eating protein also reduces your level of the hormone ghrelin, which the stomach produces and releases. Ghrelin signals to the brain when your stomach is empty and that it's time to eat. Research shows that protein also boosts levels of another hormone called peptide YY, released after eating, which contributes to feelings of fullness.[7]

The effects that protein can have on the appetite are significant.[8] In one study, increasing protein intake from 15 to 30 percent of calories helped overweight women eat 441 fewer calories each day, without even trying to restrict.[9]

Protein intake can also help stave off cravings. A food craving doesn't necessarily mean you're hungry. It's more about the brain's needing a reward than the body's needing actual energy. But the best way to deal with cravings may be to get ahead of them. And one way of doing that is to increase protein intake. I like to do this with cartons of liquid egg whites. (Before you ask: All egg products outside-the-shell are USDA pasteurized. This means they have been rapidly heated to destroy any bacteria, so further cooking is not required.) I add 8 to 12 ounces (or more) to smoothies to help liquify chopped leafy vegetables, bananas, and some frozen berries. It's an easy way to use up leftover veggies and make a midday snack that boosts my energy and increases my protein. I also keep a stash of tuna pouches near my desk—brands like StarKist and Bumble Bee now make these in an impressive array of flavors. They usually have about 15 grams of protein each; I throw some tuna on a rice cake or eat it with leftover white rice, and I feel totally satisfied.

Also important, particularly for women: People who eat more protein tend to maintain bone mass better as they age and have a much lower risk of osteoporosis and fractures. Women are at particularly high risk of osteoporosis after menopause, so eating plenty of protein, as well as staying active, is a good way to help prevent that from happening. Some research shows that protein amounts over 1.2 grams per kilogram of body weight have beneficial effects on bone mass and calcium retention.[10]

Studies also show that diets supplemented by protein levels way higher than the recommended daily allowance are especially important in people who are aging and are trying to preserve lean mass.[11] As we age, we lose muscle mass and function. This process begins at around age fifty and is said to progress at a rate of .8 percent per year. Strength declines 2 to 3 percent each year. This means that by age seventy, there's a 16 percent loss of muscle mass and a roughly 50 percent loss of strength.

Protein amounts in the range of 1.2 to 1.6 grams per kilogram of body weight have been proven effective in helping retain muscle mass among an aging population. Of course, exercise—especially strength-based resistance training—can help, too.

One way to get your daily amounts of protein is through animal sources such as meat, eggs, dairy, fish, and poultry, all of which are considered complete proteins—that is, they contain all nine essential amino acids, which are important for building new muscle and tissue, including skin and bones.

Or you can look to complete plant proteins containing all nine essential amino acids, such as soybeans (including tofu), quinoa, and chia seeds. Pea protein is a popular plant protein, and while it contains all nine amino acids, it's relatively low in one, methionine. In fact legumes such as beans, lentils, and peas, which vegetarians rely on, are often low in methionine and cysteine. Whole grains like brown rice and whole wheat bread are usually low in lysine. Vegetarians or vegans just need to be aware of these limitations and try to consume different types of incomplete proteins—for instance, eating brown rice with legumes—to ensure that they get all nine amino acids. Amino acid supplements are also available, but they aren't a protein substitute. Consumers should watch for side effects from taking too much of any specific amino acid, such as bloating or abdominal pain.

Fuel with Unsaturated Fats

Fat, while calorically dense, is also an important macronutrient as it helps the body absorb vitamins and minerals and supports cell growth. Protein gets a lot of the glory in the muscle-building story, but fat is essential, too. Testosterone, a key player in the process of building muscle, is derived largely from cholesterol. A diet rich in "good" fats elevates the body's levels of "good" cholesterol, which helps produce more growth hormone and ultimately increases the production of amino acids.

Unsaturated fats include essential fatty acids that keep cell membranes fluid, and that's important to permit nutrients to be absorbed as well as to allow your cells' waste material to be excreted. You want to have enough and the right kinds of fats. That means putting the focus on polyunsaturated and monounsaturated fats such as those found in olive oil, avocado, nuts, and seeds, and those rich in omega-3 such as eggs, fish (especially fatty fish such as salmon and mackerel), and again, nuts and seeds. Omega-3 fats are anti-inflammatory; I take omega-3 supplements every day to help guard against chronic inflammation, which plays a role in the development of many diseases.

The problem is that women have been conditioned to fear fat, believing that the ingestion of fat will make them fat. But fats help with the absorption of vitamins and nutrients. What's more, while nutritionists initially vilified saturated fat for its propensity to raise the levels of "bad" cholesterol, subsequent studies have shown that there isn't enough evidence to conclude that saturated fat leads to heart disease (though replacing saturated fat with polyunsaturated fat may indeed reduce risk).[12]

How I Eat

The sport of bodybuilding involves precise nutritional calculations that look at basal metabolic rates and carb-to-fat ratios. It involves athletes measuring out macronutrients by the gram. This is what I do when I'm preparing for a competition. But in my day-to-day life, I aim to eat well and eat consistently. My number one tip is to hit your protein amounts (1.2 to 1.6 grams per kilogram of bodyweight) and to consume protein and carbs within two hours of a workout, to help muscles recover and build.

As we've learned, most of us don't eat enough protein, and I think that making sure you are getting enough food in the form of protein helps the other macronutrients fall into place. By asking yourself if you are eating enough protein, you begin to focus on positives rather than negatives.

In general, make sure the foods are whole and cooked and not from a box, and you'll do all right. A recent analysis of 281 studies in thirty-six countries, published in the *British Medical Journal*, found that the combination of carbohydrates and fats found in so-called ultra-processed foods (UPFs) such as chips, cookies, and cakes have a "supra-addictive effect on brain reward systems," similar to addiction patterns found with cigarettes and heroin.[13]

As is true with refined carbs, when someone eats UPFs, they get a spike in dopamine, resulting in a surge of good feelings. Then they inevitably crash and crave that lost good feeling. So they want more of the UPFs. Using the same guidelines for measuring substance abuse, the researchers found that 14 percent of adults and 12 percent of children were addicted to ultra-processed foods.

UPFs are linked to obesity and chronic disease, and I feel strongly that cutting them out as much as possible is one of the best things you can do for your health, right up there with quitting smoking. These foods are extraordinarily addictive. Food companies manufacture them to be this way so that more boxes and bags are bought and sold. In a 2019 study reported in the journal *Cell Metabolism,* twenty healthy volunteers were in random order provided with meals made up of ultra-processed foods or meals made up of minimally processed foods. The meals had the same amounts of calories, sugars, fiber, fat, and carbohydrates, and participants were allowed to eat as much or as little as they wanted. Those on the ultra-processed diet ate about 500 calories more per day and gained an average of two pounds. Those on the minimally processed diet lost about that much.[14]

To put that in perspective, anywhere from 60 to 90 percent of the typical American diet is made up of UPFs, according to research. And processing removes so much *good* in food—

vitamins, minerals, fiber, and the like—while adding unnecessary ingredients like gums, fillers, and flavors.

So while you want to avoid eating UPFs whenever possible, eating like an athlete means knowing that food is something to be embraced, not something to be restricted. When I eat, I am choosing the foods that fuel my physical goals, give me energy, help me build muscle and strength, and keep me going. The building blocks for my meals are straightforward—carbs, proteins, the right fats. From these kinds of simple components, I can throw together any meal—for myself and for my family.

I reach for food because it's diverse, interesting, and tasty—and it literally keeps me alive. In terms of recipes, I have my "greatest hits," and I don't ponder diet trends or buy into food marketing. I don't get fancy with expensive oils, butters, or complicated recipes. I eat frequently—every couple of hours—and use what I have stowed away in my fridge or pantry. These days, I feel nourished, not deprived. I feel smart and empowered. I focus mainly on lean proteins like whitefish, chicken breast, and egg whites. I don't demonize carbohydrates, though I aim to eat whole ones that are minimally processed (white potatoes, sweet potatoes, brown rice), and I am careful with my fats, sticking mainly to olive oil, nut butters, and avocados.

Here are some of the ingredients that power my daily life:

Carbs (produce)	Lettuce	Apples	Cauliflower
	Tomatoes	Oranges	Celery
	Carrots	Pears	Green beans
	Bananas	Strawberries	Grapefruit
	Cucumbers	Blueberries	Lemons
	Pineapple	Blackberries	Asparagus
	Radishes	Raspberries	Potatoes
	Onions	Broccoli	Sweet potatoes
	Garlic	Brussels sprouts	
Complex carbs	Quinoa	High-fiber/sprouted breads	Multigrain cereals
	Long-grain rice	High-fiber cereal	Kamut
	Brown rice	Wheat germ	Black beans
	Spelt bread	Chickpeas	Whole-wheat pasta
	Ezekiel bread	Millet	Farro
	Steel-cut oats	Barley	Lentils
	Rolled oats		
Protein (lean)	Whitefish (cod, halibut, rockfish, etc.)	Egg whites	Lean ham
		Ground turkey (93 percent lean and above)	Shrimp
	Chicken breast (and other skinless poultry)		Shellfish
		Lean ground beef (94 percent lean and up)	Tofu
Protein (medium/higher fat)	Pork chops	Lamb chops	Salmon
	Chicken thighs/legs	Bacon	Tuna
	Stew meats	Ribs	Swordfish
	Beef	Skirt steak	Eggs

Fats	Nuts	Margarine	Seeds and seed oils
	Nut butters	Avocado	
			Coconut
	Oils	Ghee	
			Coconut butter/oil
	Salad dressing	Olives	
	Bacon drizzle	Anchovies	Mayonnaise
	Butter	Herring	

Bodybuilders weigh their food routinely to get the precise number of macronutrients down to the gram. I don't recommend this as an everyday practice, but when you're at home, it's not a bad idea to have a kitchen scale on the counter to get used to knowing what portion sizes look like. After so many years of weighing, I know what thirty-two grams of peanut butter and four ounces of cooked chicken breast look like just by eyeballing. Another good way to measure is to think about it in terms of the size of your hand:

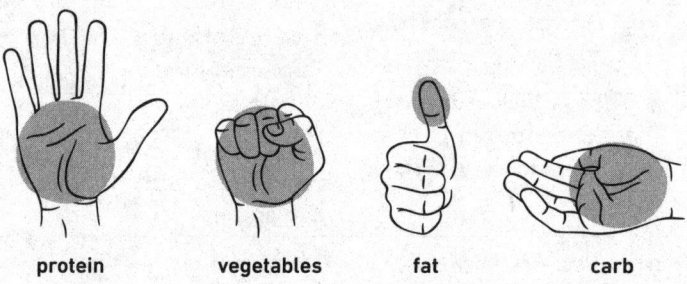

protein   vegetables   fat   carb

I can get a single tablespoon scoop to look pretty close to the pad of my thumb (which, by the way, is different from what I *once* thought a tablespoon of peanut butter looked like). And if I want to measure 3 ounces of chicken breast, then I know that's about the size of the palm of my hand, while 120 grams of cooked rice is about the size of a ball in the scoop of my hand.

Meal Planning

I don't consider myself a cook by any stretch, but I'm a damn good meal planner. Everyone has their own best way of doing things, but here's how I go about it.

1. Always keep a large green salad in the fridge.

I make a point of building up my fridge on the weekend, making sure I have enough for several big kitchen-sink salads filled with an array of my favorite vegetables, ones I know will last longer than a day or two (these aren't necessarily vegetables we think of as salad veggies—and that's okay): bok choy, chopped broccoli stems, radishes, Napa cabbage, carrots. I don't get caught up in recipes or what a salad should or shouldn't contain. Anything green goes in: celery leaves, green beans that didn't get eaten the night before, you name it. I also tend to lean on hardier vegetables that won't wilt. For example, kale, spinach, and bok choy tend to last longer than lettuces. I throw in tomatoes, cucumbers, carrots, and sliced radishes. That salad serves as a great base for all kinds of proteins and as filler for lunchtime wraps. I'll even dip into the salad just for snacking. I put it on the table at dinnertime, and everyone eats from that big, delicious bowl of mess.

2. Prep your carbs.

I like to have several carbs on hand. I prepare them once or twice a week and keep them in containers in the refrigerator. My go-tos are cooked white rice and cooked potatoes (either white or sweet potatoes, sometimes both). I usually have a few bananas on my countertop (for mixing into smoothies), and I like chopped pineapple (I buy a whole pineapple, chop it up, and stow it in a container in the fridge). For family meals, cooking, and side dishes, I always have a couple of "cooking veggies" on hand in the crisper drawer. Cauliflower, broccoli, green beans, and Brussels sprouts are safe bets. I also have two bags of nothing-added frozen veggies in the freezer in case I find myself in a pinch.

3. Plan your proteins.

On Sundays, I cook a batch of protein ahead of time. It might be chicken thrown on the grill. Maybe I'll make some turkey crumbles—a blend of ground 93 percent and 99 percent lean turkey thrown into a Crockpot with some taco seasoning and cooked slowly on low. When the kids come home from school, we have taco night (and I use the crumbles over salad, in wraps, over a sweet potato—pretty much anything). Or it might be steamed shrimp, peeled, tails removed and ready to be scooped up. I eat a lot of shrimp. I usually keep eight to ten bags of frozen shrimp around, and I thaw one out every other day. It's just easy protein and delicious over salad, cooked with some rice, or even just cold on a hot day. Once or twice a week I also eat rockfish, which is a whitefish local to my area, and I live a stone's throw from a fish market. The owner doesn't even ask me what I want anymore. When I come in, he automatically puts a fillet or two on the scale and looks at me, eyebrows raised, and I say, "Good." I also grill a package or two of chicken tenderloins—also easy protein and the kids love it—each week.

Other standards in a given week:

- **Egg whites:** I buy quarts of egg whites and make protein-packed smoothies with them. I usually combine anywhere from 8 to 12 ounces of egg whites with some banana (for carbs) and some peanut butter (for fats). I sometimes add cold-brew coffee to that and some ice. I also add egg whites to warm cereals to boost protein content. (In a pinch, I even drink some on their own, in a shaker with a little stevia and some cinnamon.) Some people balk at the notion of consuming raw egg whites, but they're flavorless, combine well with other ingredients, and are such an easy way to get protein. Again, egg whites sold in a carton are typically pasteurized, and so they are safe to eat!

- **Bone broth:** In the fall and winter months, I make this every other week. I put four or so chicken legs in a Crockpot filled with water and let them cook for the better part of a day. Once some of the liquid is gone, I throw in coarsely chopped onions, celery, and carrots and let the broth cook down even further. After about twenty-four to thirty-six hours of cooking on low, I shut the Crockpot off, strain the liquid into a large bowl, and let the broth cool in the fridge, skimming the fat off the top. Then I pour half the broth into one container for the fridge and the other half into a second container for the freezer (or to take to the office and sip on it all week). I use it as a base for all kinds of things, from my kids' ramen to soups for myself (I'll add spinach, rice, and maybe an egg if I need extra protein or fats). It's delicious and satisfying and I always have some on hand.

Once I have my proteins, starches, and salads pre-prepared, I can grab from my different containers and put together any meal in any combination. Spices and condiments are your friends: soy sauce for an East Asian flair, or Mexican spice blends to add to ground meat for a flavorful kick. I've put spicy brown mustard and pickles and ground beef over a salad and called it "hamburger salad." The name of the game is to focus on the amount of protein, be generous on the greens, keep the carbs whole and unprocessed, and go easy on the fats.

My Five-Day Sample Meal Plan

Here is a five-day sample of what my meals look like. This is not by any means prescriptive. The portion sizes, for instance, are just to give you an idea of how much I eat. The mini-meals aren't recipes or fine-dining dishes; they're quick pull-togethers based on my personal tastes (yours might be totally different). Use this section to spark ideas for your own meals; it will also enable you to see that the focus is really not on restricting. This is plenty of food. I reach for whole foods, with protein front and center, and try to keep things pretty lean. I make sure foods are kept simple, with components prepared ahead of time. The starches and proteins (crumbles, chicken breasts) are usually cooked over the weekend, and by Thursday I'll make a second batch. These are just suggestions, provided to show how I think about throwing meals together that are prepped ahead of time. And I have no problem eating the same types of foods again and again.

For those who are curious: Sometimes my family eats the same thing as me at mealtime (or a variation of the same thing); sometimes they don't. Sometimes we eat together; sometimes we don't. In general, we eat the same ingredients from the same fridge.

DAY 1

Breakfast (Meal 1): Cream of Rice: 45 grams mixed with 4 ounces egg whites and a bit of water. In the microwave, stir every 15 seconds, or on a stovetop, stir constantly with a wire whisk. Super filling and easy on the stomach. I like a couple of tablespoons of lite maple syrup on this.

Coffee (I like Coffee Mate Italian Sweet Cream creamer with mine).

Second Breakfast (Meal 2): Breakfast burrito: one egg cooked in a microwave (a stirred egg in a small bowl with a wet paper towel on top). In the last 15 seconds, I'll put a slice of Canadian bacon over the wet paper towel. When this is done, I'll throw that into a protein wrap and add some spinach leaves in there and some salsa. This makes a great little breakfast burrito.

Lunch (Meal 3): Tossed salad with 4 ounces of crumbles on top, 100 grams of cooked rice, and some chopped pickles, along with ¼ cup of salsa.

Dinner (Meal 4): Seven hard-boiled egg whites with salt and pepper.

Pre-bedtime (Meal 5): Eight to 10 ounces of liquid egg whites, a banana, a scoop of protein powder, 16 grams of peanut butter, a dash of cinnamon.

DAY 2

Breakfast (Meal 1): One egg over easy on toasted Ezekiel bread (a sprouted bread made from whole grains and legumes).

Coffee with creamer.

Second Breakfast (Meal 2): Precooked steel-cut oats with lite maple syrup.

Lunch (Meal 3): Cooked white rice, 6 ounces of cooked chicken breast, a handful of bagged spinach with ¼ cup of salsa in a protein wrap.

Dinner (Meal 4): A big tossed salad with a sweet potato, 4 to 6 ounces of meat crumbles, and low-fat feta on top with a bit of taco sauce or salsa or mustard.

Pre-bedtime (Meal 5): Two rice cakes—one spread with a tablespoon of jam, the other with a tablespoon of peanut butter.

DAY 3

Breakfast (Meal 1): An omelet made of 2 eggs, onions, and peppers (sautéed in nonstick cooking spray).

Coffee with creamer.

Second Breakfast (Meal 2): Cold-brew coffee blended with a banana, a scoop of protein powder, a tablespoon of peanut butter, and some ice.

Lunch (Meal 3): A large tossed salad with 6 ounces of thawed precooked frozen shrimp and a dressing made of 1 tablespoon of olive oil whisked with apple cider vinegar, salt, and pepper.

Dinner (Meal 4): Mashed boiled potatoes topped with 4 ounces of crumbles and some green beans (or any cooked vegetable), plus Dijon mustard.

Pre-bedtime (Meal 5): Poor man's sushi: Tuna pouch, 100 grams of cooked rice, and some crumbled seaweed on top, with soy sauce.

DAY 4

Breakfast (Meal 1): A breakfast salad of tossed greens with an egg over easy on top and salt and pepper. The yolk makes a natural dressing.

Coffee with creamer.

Second Breakfast (Meal 2): Toasted Ezekiel bread with 1 tablespoon of peanut butter.

Lunch (Meal 3): Two cups of chicken bone broth with a scoop of cooked white rice, a handful of bagged spinach, and an egg stirred in.

Dinner (Meal 4): Four ounces of slow-cooked pulled barbecued chicken breast, sautéed veggies, a scoop of rice.

Pre-bedtime (Meal 5): Six to 8 ounces of liquid egg whites, half a banana, a scoop of protein powder, ice, vanilla extract, and cinnamon.

DAY 5

Breakfast (Meal 1): Steel-cut oats with an egg over easy on top.

Second Breakfast (Meal 2): Two ounces of leftover chicken breast chopped up and added to 1 cup of bagged shredded cabbage, warm rice, and soy sauce.

Lunch (Meal 3): Six ounces of rockfish cooked in an air fryer with a spray of nonstick cooking spray, some boiled potatoes, and wilted spinach greens.

Dinner (Meal 4): Taco night, using leftover shredded crumbles, light shredded cheese, and chopped veggies plus 3 taco shells.

Pre-bedtime (Meal 5): Half a cup of nonfat Greek yogurt with a drizzle of agave nectar.

It's Okay to Trip Up

During the week, my meal prepping and planning tends to keep me on track with my nutritional intake. Where I tend to trip up is on weekends, where all the good intentions of the week can quickly fall apart. For me, this is where I've had some of my biggest challenges.

What I've learned is that I make the worst food choices when I'm happiest—relaxing, hanging out with friends and family, chilling at a restaurant or bar. Why? Because food is something that binds people together. It's a date night out, popcorn at the movies, a Christmas party with a fancy spread, or a rollicking night in the TV room with the kids and a movie. But I found that after I indulged myself I felt compelled to re-indulge, hitting a point where I was unable to stop, and this would always make me feel ill or uncomfortable afterward.

I've managed to train myself to slow down and enjoy the time, the food, the ambience, and the presence of the people I love. I eat the popcorn, but I try not to rush through the bag. I try to remind myself that I don't have to order everything on the menu including dessert. Restaurant food is laden with butters and sauces and fats, and so of course it is more delicious and more difficult to stop eating. The same is true of packaged snack foods, desserts, and alcohol. It's very hard to stop or to know when to stop.

In the end, these moments of celebration—around a birthday cake or hauls of Easter or Halloween candy, at the office party—aren't really about the food. They're about a moment and the people I'm around. I realized that when I focused on enjoying where I was and what was going on, it became less about the food, my anxiety lessened, and I was able to relax and not over-eat so much. That's key: When we feel restricted and allow ourselves a treat, it's hard to stop. Researchers call it the "what the hell" effect common among dieters:[15] The thinking is that the diet is blown, so you might as well go whole hog. And so I make sure that when I allow myself the popcorn or the birthday cake or whatever, I really don't obsess or beat myself up later. I recognize that I had a good time, I enjoyed it for what it was, and then I move on.

Staying Hydrated

Drinking water regularly does not come naturally to me, but as athletes, we need to keep our bodies hydrated. We need water to keep our body's processes in equilibrium, transporting nutrients to cells and aiding our metabolism.

Drinking water also helps increase your body's ability to burn calories, a process known as thermogenesis. During thermogenesis, your body uses energy to heat the water to body temperature, thereby burning calories. Water helps with digestion, too, breaking down food so that your body can absorb the nutrients, preventing constipation, keeping the digestive system running smoothly, and ultimately contributing to a healthier metabolism.

The U.S. National Academies of Sciences, Engineering, and Medicine has determined that an adequate daily fluid intake is about 15.5 cups (3.7 liters) of fluids a day for men and about 11.5 cups (2.7 liters) of fluids a day for women. These recommendations, by the way, include all fluids—water and other beverages and foods containing water.[16] Another benefit to fibrous fruits and vegetables is that water makes up most of their content. In fact, about 20 percent of our daily fluid intake usually comes from what we eat, and the rest from what we drink.[17]

Active individuals need even more, particularly if they're exercising in hot weather. This is especially important during the twenty-four hours prior to vigorous exercise.

To prevent dehydration and make sure your body has the fluids it needs, stick to just water—rather than other beverages—having at least one decent-size glass with each meal. You should also drink between meals as well as before, during, and after exercise. In other words, all the time! Sometimes hunger or cravings are really just dehydration. Sipping on water helps.

While I'm training, I aim to drink about 3.5 liters of pure water a day. I have a favorite water bottle that has a compartment at the top for fresh fruit, which flavors the water a bit. Remember, water doesn't necessarily need to be cold. In the winter months, I sip on hot or warm water, sometimes throwing in a piece of ginger or lemon or a tea bag of herbal tea. If I drink water cold, I'll add in a few blueberries or a sprig of mint to make it feel a little special.

As with the food I eat, the way I drink water is all part of my philosophy of not surrounding my intake with negative connotations, and instead finding ways to make it something special. I'm all about taking things from the negative column and putting them in the positive one.

People sometimes ask if I still drink alcohol, and I still do, but only on occasions such as holidays or date nights. It doesn't have the stranglehold on me that it once did. The truth is, a lot of people think of alcohol as a way to wind down, but it tends to produce a lot of chaos in the body, especially as we get older. For one thing, I find that alcohol tends to worsen my sleep—the duration of sleep tends to be shorter and the quality poorer. After I stopped drinking so much, I felt like my digestive health improved dramatically. And of course alcohol inhibits fat metabolism, which is never a great thing. Women in particular are hit harder than men when it comes to alcohol use. Women experience declining brain function faster than men. Women are at greater risk of developing alcohol-related liver diseases and are also more likely to develop mental health disorders such as anxiety and depression.

There are so many great nonalcoholic beverages to experiment with. For example, I love De Soi canned mocktails or sometimes just make my own mocktail with lime juice, grapefruit juice, and seltzer. I find that I don't need the actual ingredient of alcohol to feel like I am winding down socially.

In the end, good food and beverage are a pleasure—so much more than the instant-gratification, quick-hit processed varietals or takeout that gives you a high but ultimately makes you feel terrible afterward. There are so many wonderful foods and flavors to choose from. Take your time and explore the spice aisles or international aisles at the grocery store. You never know what new flavor or condiment you might come across. Look forward to bringing a new ingredient home or finding a way to combine foods. Another thing: Eating this way—focused on whole foods and on eating at home—also saves so much money. It's all part of the magic of fueling your body with the good stuff, which will ultimately help you build it for a longer and stronger life ahead.

EPILOGUE

I'm now training for my third season as a competitive body-builder, my first as a pro. My travel schedule this year will include a competition in Denver, Colorado, followed by one in Norfolk, Virginia, and another in Charlotte, North Carolina. I'll bring my partner and my kids and we'll make an adventure out of it. In preparation for the weeks ahead, I'm diligently following a training schedule of four to five one-hour lifting sessions a week, along with some cardio exercise, and of course the usual persnickety attention to my nutrition.

As I write this, I'm in the midst of the twelve- to sixteen-week journey that bodybuilders call prep. My visits to the gym usually begin with a warm-up stretch in the sauna. If there are other women there, I usually like to chat about anything besides work. I stay there for about ten minutes, allowing my muscles to relax and warm up. Then I hit a cardio machine (I switch up the weapon of choice on different days, to keep things interesting). I exercise for just five to seven minutes on a treadmill, rowing machine, or bike (or really whatever—sometimes it's little boxing jabs in a corner or a mini dance session in the sauna) to get the heart rate up a bit. I'll stretch. Then I course through three sets of six to eight different exercises meant to hit various muscle groups. On Mondays, that might be Bulgarian split squats, bench presses, Romanian deadlifts, chin-ups, squats, and some core work. On Tuesdays, it's a combination of different types of hip thrusts, push-ups, pistol squats, kickbacks, and chin-ups. On Wednesdays, it's more types of hip thrusts, bench presses, 45-degree hyperextensions, inverted rows, lateral raises, and hip abductions and adductions. Mind you, these aren't "kill yourself until you're sweaty and red in the face" type exercises. They are work, but they also feel steady, focused, and challenging.

At the end of the workout, I'll do about thirty minutes of required cardio (performed about five times a week, for this stage of the game). I'll typically do this at the end so as not take any energy away from the muscle-building stuff. I usually hit the stairmill machine (which mimics the feeling of climbing actual stairs). If it's a beautiful day out, I might try a long jog. Cardio is only done in the weeks before a competition, as part of my cut, to lean out and to showcase muscle.

There is a nutritional gamesmanship in these weeks, to maximize a certain look that isn't meant to last. For instance, I carb cycle on no-workout days to reduce carbs. (Fat grams on those days thankfully move up a bit.) The technique is to eliminate body fat in the weeks ahead without losing too much muscle. It's to look a certain way, but not to live a certain way.

The weekly check-ins with my coach go into extraordinary, sometimes embarrassing detail. I fill out a form every week, providing my weight for that day, but also for at least three other days of the week. I describe how my poops look and whether that's normal, how much water I'm drinking, how my workouts felt that week, whether I followed my nutrition plan, whether I'm doing any cardio, and if so, what kind of cardio I'm doing and for how many minutes. It also asks how stressed out I am on a scale from 1 to 10, and whether there is anything unusual happening in my life. I send pictures to my coach wearing a practice suit—a bikini cut similarly to a competition suit, but without the spangles. I show a front pose and a back pose. Either my partner Rick or one of my daughters takes the pictures (and teases me mercilessly). In the weeks ahead of competition, I'll attend a few posing workshops, alongside my coach's other athletes, to practice what it feels like to be on stage next to other bikini competitors. My coach will correct my form: positioning the hands, torquing the body, and standing in a way that maximizes the best attributes. Holding muscle poses in heels, while spinning around in half turns, can be excruciating, and it takes practice.

During my cutting phase, I'll inevitably lose some muscle with the fat loss. And part of me hates buying into this bikini-body idolatry. But it's short-lived. After the competition is over, I'll "reverse diet" to build my weight (and my muscle) back up from stage weight. Sometimes that's hard. I'll miss my abs. And I question myself: *Am I a hypocrite for putting a dieted version of myself on a stage to be celebrated, knowing that it's not a "real" look?*

Paulina Porizkova, the former 1980s supermodel turned champion for aging women, addressed this notion of potential hypocrisy in a recent Instagram post, where she posed in a swimsuit, admitting she felt better with a spray tan. "In getting the spray tan, I am putting out the message that a 'tan' looks better with a bikini," she says. "That tans are preferable to pale skin—although repeated tanning can actually cause physical harm."[1] She articulates discomfort with supporting a message that is not in line with her actual beliefs. (And let it be said that I'm pretty sure Paulina would look spectacular in a bikini without the spray tan! But I get it.) "I have no solution to this quandary—I'm just letting you all know that I also ping-pong between the two poles, and hope to mostly land somewhere in the middle." In being open about this quandary, she normalizes something that I think many women these days can relate to: what it means to live in a system of beauty that we can't completely escape.

It's okay to struggle with an order in which we not only exist but that has long acted as currency for us. This system has relentlessly taught us to value beauty above all else, while defining it in a very narrow way. We can cut ourselves a little slack. I think it's all right to question and struggle with it, and also to want to occupy a framework that's familiar and that works for us. I think it all just adds up to needing more representation of different kinds of beauty.

There have been inevitable bumps along the road these past few months of my life. At my place of work there have been layoffs, and I worry that my job is on the line. My car was stolen. One morning, I woke up to antisemitic slurs spray-painted on the front of our house. My older daughter refuses to smile, while the younger one refuses to sleep. Most days I feel like I'm failing as a parent. Sometimes I convince myself that everything is conspiring against me and that I've lost control. But when I have these moments, my training has taught me well. Of course there are things I can't control. But I can control myself and the choices I make. Whatever may be happening in the world and in my life, my attention to exercise, nutrition, and rest is my constant through line. It is my pact with myself.

That's not to say I don't slip up. On one occasion, while staying late at the office to finish a document, I stress-ate an old bag of Halloween candy. Another time, I was so dejected I barely made it to the gym and exercised very little once I got there. On those days, I give myself credit for showing up—and I keep showing up time and time again. There is something profound about that.

The lift—both literal and figurative—that happens in my body and my mind when I train is so powerful. My outlook on life completely changes. Things that once felt impossible now feel possible. I feel relaxed. Positive. Accomplished.

Perhaps most important, I no longer feel I am alone. In the time since I started bodybuilding in 2019, I've begun noticing a real change in the number of women present at the gym. In my early days of training, women were few and far between, my gym had a decidedly bro vibe, and I often felt like the odd one out. Now women are showing up in much larger numbers, and not just as cardio bunnies. They are lifting weights. They wear stylish ensembles—there are so many brands and options now available to them, at different price points—and they aren't afraid to show skin. They tend to be in their twenties and thirties, so I'm guessing they've been inspired by workout videos on TikTok or Instagram. They're spotting one another at the barbell rack. They are horsing around and flirting, confident. They are no longer an anomaly, there as eye candy for the men who grunt loudly. They are grunting, too. They belong there.

I've thought a lot about belonging in sports and what that means. The doors that allow us into athletic spaces are still relatively new—they haven't been open to girls and women for very long. We have had only fifty years of real, documented equality through Title IX, which aimed to level the playing field for women in both academics and sports. And there are still inequities to this day. A 2022 report by *USA Today* found that 87 percent of colleges and universities are not offering athletic opportunities to female students proportionate to enrollment, which is one of the tests of Title IX, and perhaps the clearest way that athletic programs can show compliance.[2] Educational institutions can lose their federal funding if they don't meet certain standards. We still have a long way to go.

Years ago, both of my daughters got into ice hockey. I had wanted ice hockey to be a sport that introduced them to the ice, but one in which body size or shape or their gender wouldn't be such a factor as it had been for me when I was trying to figure-skate or row for my college team. I see now I may have been too idealistic. The younger one quit hockey last year (but has found a new home in martial arts practicing self-defense). My older daughter quit the sport this summer.

So we have started lifting together. She's too young yet to be allowed into most commercial gyms, but we do little basement sessions. Her attention starts to wander after a couple of exercises, and that's okay. It lasts for all of about fifteen to twenty minutes. But she's getting the idea. And when we are doing something physical together it makes it easier for us to talk. As C. Vaile Wright, a senior director at the American Psychological Association, once told me in an interview, for some people, it's more comfortable for them to open up when they aren't face-to-face. Little distractions, mishaps, or other occurrences during physical activity create stories or laughter that fuel conversation—and make the connection between my daughter and me feel natural.

I love that I get to show her this side of my life. I want her to grow up believing it's completely normal for her mother to lift weights, to train hard, to put herself out there to compete in sports, even in her fifties. I hope that influences her to want to be a strong woman, and that she will always look to other strong women for guidance and for inspiration.

After all, it's thanks to my eldest daughter that I ever came back to my body and to athletics in the first place. If I hadn't signed her up for ice hockey—a sport where little girls haven't traditionally been welcome—I would never have run into Sara, the bodybuilder, in a little weight room at our hotel, an encounter that changed my life. My journey to bodybuilding started with looking up to another woman. Through bodybuilding, I could finally feel at home in a sport. That chance meeting with Sara revolutionized the way I think about women, strength, and our bodies, flipping a switch that led to a better, healthier, and stronger life for me.

I hope this book does the same for you.

ACKNOWLEDGMENTS

I feel grateful to have been lifted by such a diverse and lovable cast of friends, family, and allies who supported me through the four years it took to get this book on paper.

First, I would like to thank my mom, Louise, to whom this book is dedicated. Mom, you have always been my staunchest defender; my lovable, completely charming and goodhearted soul; most trusted advisor, coconspirator, coparent, and agent of fun, who has always, always, always been by my side no matter what. I love you to the moon and back. You are the strongest person I know and the shoulder I still lean on, my one call from jail, my stop-by on the way home, the voice that soothes me, and I am so lucky that you are both my neighbor and best friend. Writing this book has required many late nights and weekends that pulled me away, and I am so grateful for all your under-standing and your help—with the girls, the dog, and just about everything else.

To my brother, Carl, for having made the decision to move to DC. What a blessing to have you and your family so close. Thank you for bringing Sylvie along on all your adventures, from scouts to jiu-jitsu to all the camping trips. We love having Dahlia with us on the crazy train and we treasure her.

To my girls, my mooshkies, my great loves. Juliette and Sylvie, this book is for you. Your character and hearts are already so strong. May you continue to grow in and with the world and be wise and do good things. Don't compare yourself to anyone else. Don't think about what people want you to be. Just be you. Take up space. Eat well. Be loud. Use your noodle. Have fun. Be strong. Put yourself out there. I love you so so so much.

To their dad, Jess. Your continued friendship and support mean so much to me. I am grateful and proud that we have continued to parent these two critters together. Thank you for always being in my corner. You are valued and loved.

To my dad, Peter, who passed away before the events that led to this book were set in motion. I often wonder what he would have thought about all of it. I think he is somewhere smiling, slightly weirded out, and amused. And proud, as he always was of his kids.

To my coach, Tina Peratino, who has been through thick and thin with me, and from whom I have learned so much—not only about muscle and nutrition, but also about big-deal life stuff: that physical health isn't about just the body but also the mind and the spirit. That we can be demanding of ourselves but that it's equally important to take it easy. And to my teammates on Team CSFP, including Nancy Hurwitz, Nathalie Drexler, and of course, Sara Chiappone, who made such an impression in a dinky fitness room at a hockey rink. You just never know, sometimes, those moments that can alter your life . . .

I've had incredible colleagues and editors over the years at *The*

ACKNOWLEDGMENTS

Wall Street Journal: Rich Jaroslovsky, who hired me as his administrative assistant all those years ago, which allowed me to discover the world of journalism, and for that I am forever grateful. Larry Rout, who later hired me and became a mentor and sounding board in the years that followed. John Blanton, who made every story—and every day in the newsroom—so much better. I've actually been fortunate to have worked for, with, and alongside countless rock stars, including Edward Felsenthal, Eben Shapiro, Joanne Lipman, Hilary Stout, Tara Parker-Pope, Joann Lublin, Raju Narisetti, Bryan Gruley, Alan Murray, Marcus Brauchli, Nikhil Deogun, Jonathan Clements, Tom Herman, Laurie P. Cohen, Laurie McGinley, June Kronholz, Winston Wood, Rick Schmitt, Mary Lu Carnevale, John Hechinger, Betsy McKay, Carrie Dolan, Jennifer Levitz, and Rachel Emma Silverman, among many others. Thank you, Erin White and Lisa Bannon, for believing in my story and helping see it across the finish line.

Of course, my friends in the Washington, DC, bureau—I'm not sure what I would have done without your support: Stephanie Armour, James Grimaldi, Jack Gillum, and Kristina Peterson, among others who were there for me when I needed it the most.

A massive thank-you to Tim Martell, the executive director of the Independent Association of Publishers' Employees, who works tirelessly on behalf of employees of *The Wall Street Journal* newsroom. And to superstar attorney Stephen Z. Chertkof and his beautiful, intelligent, and warm wife, Elizabeth Cullen. I value your friendship, both of you.

This book would have not been possible without my super-agent, Todd Shuster, who saw the possibilities in my story from our very first phone call. And to Eve Claxton of Unfurl Productions, for your incredible skills as an editor, for keeping me honest, for talking me off the ledge countless times, and for being that perfect combination of drill sergeant and fairy godmother. I still hear your voice in my head. Thank you.

To the extraordinary team at Avery, for your support through and through: Isabel McCarthy, Lucia Watson, Farin Schlussel, and many others, thank you from the bottom of my heart.

Thank you to the many experts and sources cited in the book who took the time to talk with me, to share their stories and their research. Thank you, Sofia Frei, for your thoughtful readings! You are such an impressive young woman. Idan Ravin, your friendship means so much, and readers now benefit from your expertise. Maria Colacurcio, thank you for your unwavering support of my story, for sharing yours—and for the introduction to the inimitable Pattie Sellers. Pattie, I cannot thank you enough for your encouragement and friendship. This has been so damn fun. And a huge thank-you to Steve Mosko of Village Roadshow and Scott Greenstein of SiriusXM. I cannot wait to see the magic of *Lift* in other iterations!

They say it takes a village, and these people—my eclectic, loving, caring, and generous neighbors on Chesapeake Avenue—are my village: Danny and Gail Peck; Ian and Erin Delmonte; Larry and Cindy Bostian; Heather Goss and Angela An; Calvin and Annie Kee; Jonathan Harwitz and Sandhya Mehta; Amy and Tim Craig; and Kathleen and David Bartels, to name just a few. A special thanks also to the team at Gold's Gym DC Metro for your generous support, including the good people at Gold's in Silver Spring, where I train.

Thanks to the people of ImpactEleven, including Ryan Estis,

Jenny DeRosse, Ivy Gustafson, Josh Linkner, Bob Marsh, Seth Mattison, and Connor Trombley, among others. So happy to have joined the community and looking forward to many months of learning and hustle. And to my extraordinary team: Samantah Fakahany; Kamila Khasanova of On Top Strategy; Conner Krizancic of SpeakrBrand.

Finally, thank you to my *Lift* posse of incredible badass women who have supported me throughout this process—and continue to. Kamila Khasanova, thank you for your wisdom and support—I can't wait to see what we conquer next. Sam Fakahany, you are a spectacular editor and friend. Stevie Johns, I am so glad that fate allowed us to meet. I can't wait to work with you and Taylor.

A special shout-out to the ladies of the Salzman clan, who have brought me into the fold with love and warmth and supported me in this project. They include Karen Salzman-Lewis, Kassie Lewis, Debbie Smith, Laura Weeks, Eliza Salzman, and Becky Lasky.

Last but not least, to my life partner, Rick Salzman. Ricky, you make the sun shine. I have learned so much from you—about how to live joyfully, how to appreciate the micro moments, and how to really value the stuff that matters and to let go of what doesn't. Life is just better—a little lighter and brighter—with you in it. Your smile and those twinkling blue-green eyes make me melt. Your love and unwavering support mean everything. I feel so lucky to be able to share my life with you.

Let's keep going.

NOTES

Introduction

1. "Dopamine," Health Direct, August 2023, https://www.health direct.gov.au/dopamine.
2. "What Is Noradrenaline?," Mental Health America, https://mha national.org/what-noradrenaline#24.
3. "Women May Realize Health Benefits of Regular Exercise More Than Men," National Heart, Lung, and Blood Institute news release, February 19, 2024, https://www.nhlbi.nih.gov/news/2024/women-may-realize-health-benefits-regular-exercise-more-men.
4. "The Unique Benefits of Strength Training for Women," The Science of Health, University Hospitals, April 29, 2024, https://www.uhhospitals.org/blog/articles/2024/04/the-unique-benefits-of-strength-training-for-women.
5. Darragh O'Sullivan et al., "Effects of Resistance Exercise Training on Depressive Symptoms Among Young Adults: A Randomized Controlled Trial," *Psychiatry Research* 326 (2023): 115322, https://doi.org/10.1016/j.psychres.2023.115322.
6. Haruki Momma et al., "Muscle-Strengthening Activities Are Associated with Lower Risk and Mortality in Major Non-Communicable Diseases: A Systematic Review and Meta-Analysis of Cohort Studies," *British Journal of Sports Medicine* 56, no. 13 (2022): 755–63, https://bjsm.bmj.com/content/56/13/755.

7. Brian Uzzi, "Research: Men and Women Need Different Kinds of Networks to Succeed," *Harvard Business Review*, February 25, 2019, https://hbr.org/2019/02/research-men-and-women-need-different-kinds-of-networks-to-succeed.

8. Alison A. Macintosh, Ron Pinhasi, and Jay T. Stock, "Prehistoric Women's Manual Labor Exceeded That of Athletes Through the First 5500 Years of Farming in Central Europe," *Science Advances* 3, no. 11 (2017): eaao3893, https://www.science.org/doi/10.1126/sciadv.aao3893.

9. Brian Huchel-Purdue, "Women's Sports Still Get 'Bland' Coverage," *Futurity*, March 24, 2021, https://www.futurity.org/womens-sports-coverage-2537412-2/.

10. Cheryl Cooky, "One and Done: The Long Eclipse of Women's Televised Sports, 1989–2019," *Communication & Sport* 9, no. 3 (2021): 347–71, https://journals.sagepub.com/doi/full/10.1177/21674795211003524.

Chapter 1: The Story of Skinny

1. Meghan Casserly, "Can Bethenny Crack a Billion?," *Forbes*, May 19, 2011, https://www.forbes.com/2011/05/17/celebrity-100-11-bethenny-frankel-skinnygirl-bravo-money-makers.html?sh=44f68030430e.

2. Emily Burack, "Read America Ferrera's Powerful Monologue in *Barbie*," *Town & Country*, August 5, 2023, https://www.townandcountrymag.com/leisure/arts-and-culture/a44725030/america-ferrera-barbie-full-monologue-transcript/.

3. Garabed Eknoyan, "A History of Obesity, or How What Was Good Became Ugly and Then Bad," *Advances in Chronic Kidney Disease* 13, no. 4 (2006): 421–27, https://pubmed.ncbi.nlm.nih.gov/17045228/.

4. Eknoyan, "A History of Obesity."

5. "How Do We Know Baroque Art Depicted Obese Ladies Because of a Different Idea of Beauty?," History Stack Exchange, https://history.stackexchange.com/questions/50562/how-do-we-know-baroque-art-depicted-obese-ladies-because-of-a-different-ideal-of.

6. Mimi Matthews, "Victorian Fat Shaming: Harsh Words on Weight from the 19th Century," *Mimi Matthews* (blog), April 25, 2016, https://www.mimimatthews.com/2016/04/25/victorian-fat-shaming-harsh-words-on-weight-from-the-19th-century/.

7. Emily Clark, "Sylvester Graham: Progressive Advocate for Healthy Living," ConnecticutHistory.org, October 1, 2022, https://connecticuthistory.org/sylvester-graham-progressive-advocate-for-healthy-living/.

8. Sylvester Graham, *Treatise on Bread, and Bread-Making* (Boston: Light & Stearns, 1837), v; Lisa Kingsley, "The Seesawing History of Fad Diets," *Smithsonian Magazine*, February 27, 2023, https://www.smithsonianmag.com/innovation/the-seesawing-history-of-fad-diets-180981586/.

9. Hillel Schwartz, *Never Satisfied: A Cultural History of Diets, Fantasies, and Fat* (New York: Free Press, 1986).

10. Schwartz, *Never Satisfied*.

11. "Overview," *The Gibson Girl's America: Drawings by Charles Dana Gibson* (exhibition), Library of Congress, https://www.loc.gov/exhibits/gibson-girls-america/overview.html.

12. "Achieving the Gibson Girls' Silhouette: It's All About the Padding," *Recollections* (blog), August 17, 2021, https://recollections.biz/blog/achieving-the-gibson-girl-s-silhouette/.

13. "The Gibson Girl as the 'New Woman,'" *The Gibson Girl's America: Drawings by Charles Dana Gibson* (exhibition), Library of Congress, https://www.loc.gov/exhibits/gibson-girls-america/the-gibson-girl-as-the-new-woman.html.

14. Naomi Wolf, *The Beauty Myth: How Images of Beauty Are Used Against Women* (New York: William Morrow, 1991).

15. Brett Silverstein and Deborah Perlick, *The Cost of Competence: Why Inequality Causes Depression, Eating Disorders, and Illness in Women* (New York: Oxford University Press, 1995).

16. Silverstein and Perlick, *The Cost of Competence*.

17. Gina Kolata, "Chubby Gets a Second Look," *New York Times*, November 11, 2007, https://www.nytimes.com/2007/11/11/weekinreview/11kolata.html.

18. Silverstein and Perlick, *The Cost of Competence*.

19. David Kamp, "Whether True or False, a Real Stretch," *New York Times*, December 30, 2008, https://www.nytimes.com/2008/12/31/dining/31diam.html.

20. Silverstein and Perlick, *The Cost of Competence*.

21. *The Journal* (New York [N.Y.]), May 19, 1896, https://www.loc.gov/resource/sn84031792/1896-05-19/ed-1/.

22. Silverstein and Perlick, *The Cost of Competence*.

23. "Lulu Hunt Peters," Wikipedia, https://en.wikipedia.org/wiki/Lulu_Hunt_Peters.

24. Brett Silverstein et al., "The Role of the Mass Media in Promoting a Thin Standard of Bodily Attractiveness for Women," *Sex Roles: A Journal of Research* 14 (1986): 519–32, https://link.springer.com/article/10.1007/BF00287452.

25. "Weight and Slimness Advertisements," Digital History—Histoire Numérique, https://omeka.uottawa.ca/jmccutcheon/exhibits/show/american-women-in-tobacco-adve/weight-and-slimness-advertisem.

26. Penny Travers, "Chart Shows Shocking Change in Clothing Sizes," *Good Housekeeping*, August 17, 2015, https://www.goodhousekeeping.com/uk/fashion-beauty/a556302/chart-shows-shocking-change-in-clothing-sizes/.

27. Kate Hardcastle, "Marilyn Monroe's Dress Size Myth: Why Fashion Must Size Up," *Forbes*, July 7, 2021, https://www.forbes.com/sites/katehardcastle/2021/07/07/marilyn-monroes-dress-size-myth-why-fashion-must-size-up/.

28. David M. Garner et al., "Cultural Expectations of Thinness in Women," *Psychological Reports* 47, no. 2 (1980): 483–91, https://journals.sagepub.com/doi/10.2466/pr0.1980.47.2.483.

29. "The Dove Case: Marketing Self-Acceptance," *Ikana Business Review*, March 3, 2024, https://ikanabusinessreview.com/2024/03/03/the-dove-case-marketing-self-acceptance/.

30. Doris G. Bazzini et al., "How Healthy Are Health Magazines? A Comparative Content Analysis of Cover Captions and Images of *Women's* and *Men's Health* Magazine," *Sex Roles: A Journal of Research* 72 (2015): 198–210, https://psych.appstate.edu/sites/psych.appstate.edu/files/howhealthyarehealthmagazines.pdf.

31. Cathaleen Chen, "'It's Not Been Enough to Carry the Day': Why the Victoria's Secret Rebrand Is Over," CNN Style, October 17, 2023, https://www.cnn.com/style/why-victorias-secret-is-bringing-sexy-back-bof/index.html.

32. Kaarin Vembar, "M.M.LaFleur Pulls Back on Plus-Size Apparel," Retail Dive, February 19, 2020, https://www.retaildive.com/news/mmlafleur-pulls-back-on-plus-size-apparel/572491/.

33. Elizabeth Endicott, "Your Clothes Were Never Meant to Fit You," *New York Times*, August 15, 2023, https://www.nytimes.com/2023/08/15/opinion/clothes-plus-size-women.html.

34. Jonel Aleccia, "Drug Used in Diabetes Treatment Mounjaro Helped Dieters Shed 60 Pounds, Study Finds," Associated Press, October 16, 2023, https://apnews.com/article/mounjaro-obesity-weight-loss-tirzepatide-ac4151fdfcd6ac17f502d1a14af4fff5.

35. Hannah Yasharoff, "Jimmy Kimmel Joked About Ozempic at the Oscars. We Need to Actually Talk About It," *USA Today*, March 13, 2023, https://www.usatoday.com/story/life/health-wellness/2023/03/13/ozempic-sweeping-hollywood-celebrities-weight-loss/11428801002/.

36. Danielle Pergament, "Kim Kardashian and I Analyzed Each Other's Faces," *Allure*, August 2022, https://www.allure.com/story/kim-kardashian-cover-interview-august-2022.

37. Dan Heching, "Amy Schumer Slams Other Stars for 'Lying' About Being on Ozempic," CNN Entertainment, June 11, 2023, https://www.cnn.com/2023/06/10/entertainment/amy-schumer-ozempic/index.html.

38. Toyin Owoseje, "Weight Loss, Motherhood and the Magazine Quiz That Made Her Rethink Her Marriage—What We Learned from Adele's Oprah Interview," CNN Entertainment, November 15, 2021, https://www.cnn.com/2021/11/15/entertainment/adele-oprah-what-we-learned-scli-intl/index.html.

39. Elizabeth Leonard, "Oprah Winfrey Reveals She Uses Weight-Loss Medication as a 'Maintenance Tool': 'I'm Absolutely Done with the Shaming,'" *People*, December 14, 2023, https://people.com/oprah-winfrey-reveals-weight-loss-medication-exclusive-8414552.

40. Michael T. Owyang and E. Katarina Vermann, "Worth Your Weight? Re-examining the Link Between Obesity and Wages," Federal Reserve Bank of St. Louis, October 1, 2011, https://www.stlouisfed.org/publications/regional-economist/october-2011/worth-your-weight-reexamining-the-link-between-obesity-and-wages

41. Frances Bozsik et al., "Thin Is In? Think Again: The Rising Importance of Muscularity in the Thin Ideal Female Body," *Sex Roles: A Journal of Research* 79 (2018): 609–15, https://doi.org/10.1007/s11199-017-0886-0.

42. Bozsik et al., "Thin Is In? Think Again."

Chapter 2: She's a Brick House

1. Alison A. Macintosh, Ron Pinhasi, and Jay T. Stock, "Prehistoric Women's Manual Labor Exceeded That of Athletes Through the First 5500 Years of Farming in Central Europe," *Science Advances* 3, no. 11 (2017): eaao3893, https://www.science.org/doi/10.1126/sciadv.aao3893.

2. Cara Ocobock, "The Theory That Men Evolved to Hunt and Women Evolved to Gather Is Wrong," *Scientific American*, November 2023, https://www.scientificamerican.com/article/the-theory-that-men-evolved-to-hunt-and-women-evolved-to-gather-is-wrong1/.

3. Sarah Lacy and Cara Ocobock, "Woman the Hunter: The Archaeological Evidence," *American Anthropologist* 126, no. 1 (2024): 19–31, https://anthrosource.onlinelibrary.wiley.com/doi/10.1111/aman.13914.

4. Abigail Anderson et al., "The Myth of Man the Hunter: Women's Contribution to the Hunt Across Ethnographic Contexts," *PLoS ONE* 18, no. 6 (2023): e0287101, https://journals.plos.org/plosone/article?id=10.1371/journal.pone.0287101.

5. Meilan Solly, "Researchers Reaffirm Remains in Viking Tomb Belonged to a Woman," *Smithsonian Magazine*, February 21, 2019, https://www.smithsonianmag.com/smart-news/researchers-reaffirm-famed-ancient-viking-warrior-was-biologically-female-180971541/.

6. Carly Cassella, "Scientists Have Proven That the 'Disputed' Female Viking Warrior Really Did Exist," *Science Alert*, February 20, 2019, https://www.sciencealert.com/researchers-double-down-on -contentious-study-showing-viking-women-warriors-existed.

7. R. J. Maughan et al., "Endurance Capacity of Untrained Males and Females in Isometric and Dynamic Muscular Contractions," *European Journal of Applied Physiology and Occupational Physiology* 55, no. 4 (1986): 395–400, https://pubmed.ncbi.nlm.nih.gov/375 8040/.

8. Emma Cowley et al., "'Invisible Sportswomen': The Sex Data Gap in Sport and Exercise Science Research," *Women in Sport and Physical Activity Journal* 29, no. 2 (2021): 1–6, https://www .researchgate.net/publication/354739161_Invisible_Sports women_The_Sex_Data_Gap_in_Sport_and_Exercise_Science _Research.

9. Thomas Beltrame, Rodrigo Villar, and Richard L. Hughson, "Sex Differences in the Oxygen Delivery, Extraction, and Uptake During Moderate-Walking Exercise Transition," *Applied Physiology, Nutrition, and Metabolism* 42, no. 9 (2017): 994–1000, https://doi .org/10.1139/apnm-2017-0097.

10. Washington Post Live, "Transcript: Leveling the Playing Field with Clara Wu Tsai," *Washington Post*, https://www.washington post.com/washington-post-live/2023/11/06/transcript-leveling -playing-field-with-clara-wu-tsai/.

11. Holly Silvers-Granelli, "Why Female Athletes Injure Their ACL's More Frequently? What Can We Do to Mitigate Their Risk?," *International Journal of Sports Physical Therapy* 16, no. 4 (2021): 971–77, https://www.ncbi.nlm.nih.gov/pmc/articles/PMC8329328/.

12. Katharine Sanderson and *Nature*, "Why Sports Concussions Are Worse for Women," *Scientific American*, September 23, 2021, https:// www.scientificamerican.com/article/why-sports-concussions -are-worse-for-women/.

13. David Dare and Scott Rodeo, "Mechanisms of Post-Traumatic Osteoarthritis After ACL Injury," *Current Rheumatology Reports* 16, no. 10 (2014): 448, https://pubmed.ncbi.nlm.nih.gov/25182676/.

14. Canadian Women & Sport, *The Rally Report: Encouraging Action to Improve Sport for Women and Girls*, June 2020, https://womenand sport.ca/resources/research-insights/rally-report/.

15. Wu Tsai Human Performance Alliance, https://www.salk.edu/wu -tsai-human-performance-alliance/.

16. Louise Høeg et al., "Higher Intramuscular Triacylglycerol in Women Does Not Impair Insulin Sensitivity and Proximal Insulin Signaling," *Journal of Applied Physiology* 107, no. 3 (2009): 824–31, https://pubmed.ncbi.nlm.nih.gov/19574502/.

17. Dan Ketchum, "Is There a Difference Between Male and Female Muscles?," Livestrong, https://www.livestrong.com/article/355987 -female-male-muscles/.

18. Yannick Molgat-Seon, Carli M. Peters, and A. William Sheel, "Sex-Differences in the Human Respiratory System and Their Impact on Resting Pulmonary Function and the Integrative Response to Exercise," *Current Opinion in Physiology* 6 (2018): 21–27, https:// www.sciencedirect.com/science/article/abs/pii/S2468867318 300506; Joseph F. Welch et al., "Sex Differences in Diaphragmatic Fatigue: The Cardiovascular Response to Inspiratory Resistance," *Journal of Physiology* 596, no. 17 (2018): 4017–32, https://www.ncbi .nlm.nih.gov/pmc/articles/PMC6117572/.

19. Rachel Chamberlain, "The Female Athlete Triad: Recommenda-tions for Management," *American Family Physician* 97, no. 8 (2018): 499–502, https://www.aafp.org/pubs/afp/issues/2018/0415/p499 .html.

20. Carly Cassella, "One of the Biggest Hunter-Gatherers Myths Is Fi-nally Getting Debunked," *Science Alert*, November 22, 2023, https:// www.sciencealert.com/one-of-the-biggest-hunter-gatherers -myths-is-finally-getting-debunked.

21. Sandra K. Hunter, "The Relevance of Sex Differences in Perfor-mance Fatigability," *Medicine & Science in Sports & Exercise* 48, no. 11 (2016): 2247–56, https://pubmed.ncbi.nlm.nih.gov/27015385/.

22. "Life Expectancy of the World Population," worldometer, https:// worldostats.com/life-expectancy-by-country-2024/#google_ vignette.

23. Katherine Schaeffer, "U.S. Centenarian Population Is Projected to Quadruple over the Next 30 Years," Pew Research Center, January 9, 2024, https://www.pewresearch.org/short-reads/2024/01/09/us -centenarian-population-is-projected-to-quadruple-over-the -next-30-years/.

24. World Supercentenarian Rankings List, Gerontology Research Group, Dr. Coles' Supercentenarian Institute, https://www.grg -supercentenarians.org/world-supercentenarian-rankings-list/.

25. Human Mortality Database, https://www.mortality.org/.

26. Edward J. Masoro and Steven N. Austad, eds., *Handbook of the Biology of Aging*, 6th ed. (Boston: Elsevier Academic Press, 2006).

27. Steven N. Austad and Andrzej Bartke, "Sex Differences in Longevity and in Responses to Anti-Aging Interventions: A Mini-Review," *Gerontology* 62, no. 1 (2015): 40–46, https://pubmed.ncbi.nlm.nih .gov/25968226/.

28. Shelley E. Taylor et al., "Biobehavioral Responses to Stress in Females: Tend-and-Befriend, Not Fight-or-Flight," *Psychological Review* 107, no. 3 (2000): 411–29, https://taylorlab.psych.ucla.edu/wp -content/uploads/sites/5/2014/10/2000_Biobehavioral-responses -to-stress-in-females_tend-and-befriend.pdf.

Chapter 3: Lift Heavy Things

1. "How Can Strength Training Build Healthier Bodies as We Age?," National Institute on Aging, June 30, 2022, https://www.nia.nih .gov/news/how-can-strength-training-build-healthier-bodies -we-age.

2. Elena Volpi, Reza Nazemi, and Satoshi Fujita, "Muscle Tissue Changes with Aging," *Current Opinion in Clinical Nutrition & Metabolic Care* 7, no. 4 (2004): 405–10, https://www.ncbi.nlm.nih.gov /pmc/articles/PMC2804956/.

3. "Osteoporosis: What You Need to Know as You Age," Johns Hopkins Medicine Health, https://www.hopkinsmedicine.org/health /conditions-and-diseases/osteoporosis/osteoporosis-what-you -need-to-know-as-you-age.

4. "Slowing Bone Loss with Weight-Bearing Exercise," Harvard Health Publishing, April 11, 2021, https://www.health.harvard.edu/staying -healthy/slowing-bone-loss-with-weight-bearing-exercise.

5. "Slowing Bone Loss with Weight-Bearing Exercise."

6. Mayo Clinic Staff, "The Reality of Menopause Weight Gain," Mayo Clinic, July 8, 2023, https://www.mayoclinic.org/healthy -lifestyle/womens-health/in-depth/menopause-weight-gain/art -20046058.

7. Mayo Clinic Staff, "Metabolism and Weight Loss: How You Burn Calories," Mayo Clinic, October 8, 2022, https://www.mayoclinic .org/healthy-lifestyle/weight-loss/in-depth/metabolism/art -20046508.

8. Lorne David Opler, "Your Brain on Barbells: Could Strength Training Help Improve Your Mood?," *Washington Post*, September 2, 2020, https://www.washingtonpost.com/lifestyle/wellness/weightlift ing-depression-anxiety-help/2020/09/01/d1036794-e882-11ea-bc79 -834454439a44_story.html.

9. Brett R. Gordon et al., "Association of Efficacy of Resistance Exercise Training with Depressive Symptoms: Meta-Analysis and Meta-Regression Analysis of Random Clinical Trials," *JAMA Psychiatry* 75, no. 6 (2018): 566–76, https://pubmed.ncbi.nlm.nih.gov/29800984/.

10. Lisa Weinberg et al., "A Single Bout of Resistance Exercise Can Enhance Episodic Memory Performance," *Acta Psychologica* 153 (2014): 13–19, https://www.sciencedirect.com/science/article/abs /pii/S0001691814001577.

11. Edward Laskowski, interview with the author, December 23, 2020.

12. Jane Lancaster, "'As Near to Flying as One Gets Outside a Circus': Charlotte Perkins Gilman and the Providence Ladies' Sanitary Gymnasium, 1881–1884," Small State Big History, http://small statebighistory.com/as-near-to-flying-as-one-gets-outside-a -circus-charlotte-perkins-gilman-and-the-providence-ladies -sanitary-gymnasium-1881-1884/.

13. Brad Kelly, "The Original Girl Gone Strong: Abbye 'Pudgy' Stockton," GirlsGoneStrong.com, https://www.girlsgonestrong.com/blog

/articles/the-original-girl-gone-strong-abbye-pudgy-stockton/; Pudgy and Les Stockton Collection, H. J. Lutcher Stark Center for Physical Culture and Sports, https://starkcenter.org/research/col lections/pudgy-and-les-stockton-collection/.

14. Associated Press, "Abbye Stockton, 88, Weight-Lifting Pioneer, Dies," *New York Times*, July 10, 2006, https://www.nytimes.com /2006/07/10/sports/10stockton.html.

15. Dennis McLellan, "Obituaries: Weightlifter Abbye 'Pudgy' Stockton, 88," *Washington Post*, July 2, 2006, https://www.washington post.com/archive/local/2006/07/03/weightlifter-abbye-pudgy -stockton-88/58b9e296-19ed-4df9-9f83-6037f1645800/.

16. Dennis McLellan, "Abbye Stockton, 88: Weightlifter Elevated the Status of Women's Fitness," *Los Angeles Times*, June 30, 2006, https://www.latimes.com/archives/la-xpm-2006-jun-30-me -stockton30-story.html

17. Jennifer Harlan, "The Long and Surprising History of Roller Derby," *New York Times*, July 26, 2019, https://www.nytimes.com/2019/07 /26/sports/roller-derby-history-photos.html.

18. Harlan, "The Long and Surprising History of Roller Derby."

19. Gay Talese, "It's a Wonderful Whirl to Gerry," *New York Times*, October 10, 1958, https://www.nytimes.com/1958/10/10/archives /its-a-wonderful-whirl-to-gerry-miss-murray-is-her-old-madcap -self.html.

20. Richard Sandomir, "Gerry Murray, Stalwart Roller Derby Star, Dies at 98," *New York Times*, August 15, 2019, https://www.ny times.com/2019/08/15/sports/gerry-murray-dead.html.

21. Jessica Strübel and Trent A. Petrie, "'Bout Time! Renegotiating the Body in Roller Derby," *Sex Roles: A Journal of Research* 74, no. 7–8 (2016): 347–60, https://doi.org/10.1007/s11199-015-0490-0.

22. Jessica Strübel, interview with the author, January 2, 2021.

23. "Gorgeous Ladies of Wrestling," Pro Wrestling Wiki, http:// prowrestling.fandom.com/wiki/Gorgeous_Ladies_of_Wrestling.

24. "Gorgeous Ladies of Wrestling."

25. Carly Mensch, interview with the author, January 25, 2024.

Chapter 4: Aging Beastfully

1. Nora Ephron, *I Feel Bad About My Neck: And Other Thoughts on Being a Woman* (New York: Knopf, 2006).

2. "Menopause," Cleveland Clinic, June 24, 2024, https://my.cleveland clinic.org/health/diseases/21841-menopause; "Perimenopause," Cleveland Clinic, August 8, 2024, https://my.clevelandclinic.org /health/diseases/21608-perimenopause.

3. Cassandra Roeca, Zain Al-Safi, and Nanette Santoro, "The Post-menopausal Women," National Library of Medicine Endotext, August 31, 2018, https://www.ncbi.nlm.nih.gov/books/NBK279131/.

4. "Preserve Your Muscle Mass," Staying Healthy, Harvard Health Publishing, February 19, 2016, https://www.health.harvard.edu /staying-healthy/preserve-your-muscle-mass.

5. Lex B. Verdijk et al., "Satellite Cells in Human Skeletal Muscle; from Birth to Old Age," *Age* (Dordr) 36, no. 2 (2014): 545–47, https://pubmed.ncbi.nlm.nih.gov/24122288/.

6. Meng-Xia Ji and Qi Yu, "Primary Osteoporosis in Postmeno-pausal Women," *Chronic Diseases and Translational Medicine* 1, no. 1 (2015): 9–13, https://www.ncbi.nlm.nih.gov/pmc/articles/PMC 5643776/.

7. "Strength Training Builds More Than Muscles," Staying Healthy, Harvard Health Publishing, January 16, 2024, https://www.health .harvard.edu/staying-healthy/strength-training-builds-more -than-muscles.

8. "Slowing Bone Loss with Weight-Bearing Exercise," Staying Healthy, Harvard Health Publishing, April 11, 2021, https://www .health.harvard.edu/staying-healthy/slowing-bone-loss-with -weight-bearing-exercise.

9. Larry Tucker, interview with the author, June 16, 2023.

10. Larry A. Tucker et al., "Effect of Two Jumping Programs on Hip Bone Density in Premenopausal Women: A Randomized Con-trolled Trial," *American Journal of Health Promotion* 29, no. 3 (2015): 158–64, https://pubmed.ncbi.nlm.nih.gov/24460005/.

11. Jacques P. Brown et al., "Mortality in Older Adults Following a Fragility Fracture: Real-World Retrospective Matched-Cohort Study in Ontario," *BMC Musculoskeletal Disorders* 22, no. 1 (2021):

105, https://bmcmusculoskeletdisord.biomedcentral.com/articles/10.1186/s12891-021-03960-z.

12. Edward Laskowski, interview with the author, December 23, 2020.

13. Jamie Bartosch, "Why Am I Gaining Weight So Fast During Menopause? And Will Hormone Therapy Help?," UChicago Medicine, April 25, 2023, https://www.uchicagomedicine.org/forefront/womens-health-articles/2023/april/menopause-weight-gain-hormone-therapy.

14. N. Salari et al., "Global Prevalence of Sleep Disorders During Menopause: A Meta-Analysis," *Sleep and Breathing* 27 (2023): 1883–97, https://www.ncbi.nlm.nih.gov/pmc/articles/PMC9996569/.

15. "Fact Sheet: Sleep During the Menopause Transition," https://www.swanstudy.org/wps/wp-content/uploads/2023/04/SWAN-Fact-Sheets-Sleep.pdf.

16. Christopher E. Kline et al., "Consistently High Sports/Exercise Activity Is Associated with Better Sleep Quality, Continuity and Depth in Midlife Women: The SWAN Sleep Study," *Sleep* 36, no. 9 (2013): 1279–88, https://www.ncbi.nlm.nih.gov/pmc/articles/PMC3738036/.

17. "Pumping Iron May Improve Sleep More Than Cardio Workouts," Iowa State University News Service, March 3, 2022, https://www.news.iastate.edu/news/2022/03/03/resistance-exercise-sleep.

18. Séverine Lamon et al., "The Effect of Acute Sleep Deprivation on Skeletal Muscle Protein Synthesis and the Hormonal Environment," *Physiological Reports* 9, no. 1 (2021): e14660, https://www.ncbi.nlm.nih.gov/pmc/articles/PMC7785053/.

19. "What to Know About Sleep Deprivation," Medical News Today, July 16, 2024, https://www.medicalnewstoday.com/articles/307334.

20. Wendy Suzuki, "The Brain-Changing Benefits of Exercise," TEDWomen 2017, November 2017, https://www.ted.com/talks/wendy_suzuki_the_brain_changing_benefits_of_exercise?subtitle=en.

21. Rebecca C. Thurston, "Cognition and the Menopausal Transition: Is Perception Reality?," *Menopause* 20, no. 12 (2013): 1231–32, https://journals.lww.com/menopausejournal/Citation/2013/12000/Cognition_and_the_menopausal_transition___is.3.aspx.

22. Suzuki, "The Brain-Changing Benefits of Exercise."

23. Todd Hollingshead, "High Levels of Exercise Linked to Nine Years of Less Aging (at the Cellular Level)," *BYU News*, May 10, 2017, https://news.byu.edu/news/high-levels-exercise-linked-nine-years-less-aging-cellular-level.

24. Selene Yeager, host, *Hit Play Not Pause*, podcast, episode 87, "Better Brain Health with Louisa Nicola," Feisty Media, June 22, 2022, https://livefeisty.com/podcasts/87-better-brain-health-with-louisa-nicola-episode-87/.

25. Avery Faigenbaum, interview with the author, March 9, 2021.

26. Centers for Disease Control and Prevention, "Prevalence of Obesity Among Children and Adolescents in the United States and Canada," CDC, accessed December 8, 2024, https://www.cdc.gov/nchs/data/hestat/obesity_child_15_16/obesity_child_15_16.htm.

27. James S. Fell, "Go Ahead, Let Those Kids Lift Weights," *Los Angeles Times*, January 10, 2011, https://www.latimes.com/archives/la-xpm-2011-jan-10-la-he-kids-weightlifting-20110110-story.html.

28. CJ Del Balso, interview with the author, June 1, 2023.

29. *Change It Up! What Girls Say About Redefining Leadership*, A Report from the Girl Scout Research Institute, https://www.girlscouts.org/content/dam/girlscouts-gsusa/forms-and-documents/about-girl-scouts/research/change_it_up_executive_summary_english.pdf.

30. Tara Sophia Mohr, "Why Women Don't Apply for Jobs Unless They're 100% Qualified," *Harvard Business Review*, August 25, 2014, https://hbr.org/2014/08/why-women-dont-apply-for-jobs-unless-theyre-100-qualified.

31. Christine L. Exley and Judd B. Kessler, "The Gender Gap in Self-Promotion," National Bureau of Economic Research, Working Paper 26345, https://www.nber.org/system/files/working_papers/w26345/revisions/w26345.rev0.pdf.

32. EY Global, "Why a Female Athlete Should Be Your Next Leader," https://www.ey.com/en_au/athlete-programs/why-a-female-athlete-should-be-your-next-leader.

33. Ellen Galinsky, interview with the author, October 17, 2024.

Chapter 5: The Mental Game

1. Sabina B. Gesell, Eric Tesdahl, and Eileen Ruchman, "The Distribution of Physical Activity in an After-School Program," *Pediatrics* 129, no. 6 (2012): 1064–71, https://www.ncbi.nlm.nih.gov/pmc/articles/PMC3362907/#:~:text=Main%20Findings, friends%2C%20 although%20other%20studies%20have.

Chapter 6: Building Your Routine

1. Jaqueline Santos Silva Lopes et al., "Effects of Training with Elastic Resistance Versus Conventional Resistance on Muscular Strength: A Systematic Review and Meta-Analysis," *SAGE Open Medicine* 7 (2019): 2050312119831116, https://www.ncbi.nlm.nih.gov/pmc/articles/PMC6383082/.

2. Xinhong Liu, "Effects of Different Resistance Exercise Forms on Body Composition and Muscle Strength in Overweight and/or Obese Individuals," *Frontiers in Physiology* 12 (2022): 791999, https://www.frontiersin.org/journals/physiology/articles/10.3389/fphys.2021.791999/full; "How Effective Are Resistance Bands for Strength Training?," Cleveland Clinic, May 4, 2022, https://health.clevelandclinic.org/should-you-try-resistance-bands-for-strength-training.

3. Jason P. Lake and Mike A. Lauder, "Kettlebell Swing Training Improves Maximal and Explosive Strength," *Journal of Strength and Conditioning Research* 26, no. 8 (2012): 2228–33, https://journals.lww.com/nsca-jscr/fulltext/2012/08000/kettlebell_swing_training_improves_maximal_and.28.aspx.

4. "Timing and Dosage for Drinking Coffee Before a Workout," Healthline, March 30, 2021, https://www.healthline.com/nutrition/coffee-before-workout#timing-dosage.

5. J. D. MacDougall et al., "The Time Course for Elevated Muscle Protein Synthesis Following Heavy Resistance Exercise," *Canadian Journal of Applied Physiology* 20, no. 4 (1995): 480–86, https://pubmed.ncbi.nlm.nih.gov/8563679/.

6. M. Dattilo et al., "Sleep and Muscle Recovery: Endocrinological and Molecular Basis for a New and Promising Hypothesis," *Med*

Hypotheses 77, no. 2 (2011): 220–22, https://doi.org/10.1016/j.mehy
.2011.04.017.

7. Jennifer Schwartz and Richard D. Simon Jr., "Sleep Extension Improves Serving Accuracy: A Study with College Varsity Tennis Players," *Physiology & Behavior* 151 (2015): 541–44, https://www
.sciencedirect.com/science/article/abs/pii/S0031938415300895.

8. Michelle Brandt, "Snooze You Win? It's True for Achieving Hoop Dreams, Says Study," Stanford Medicine News Center, June 30, 2011, https://med.stanford.edu/news/all-news/2011/07/snooze-you
-win-its-true-for-achieving-hoop-dreams-says-study.html.

9. Hui Shen, Meijuan Chen, and Donghong Cui, "Biological Mechanism Study of Meditation and Its Application in Mental Disorders," *General Psychiatry* 33, no. 4 (2020): e100214, https://doi.org/10.1136
/gpsych-2020-100214.

10. Elizabeth Bernstein, "Stressed Out, Anxious or Sad? Try Meditating," *Wall Street Journal*, December 4, 2017, https://www.wsj.com
/articles/anxious-sad-or-grumpy-try-meditating-1512404519.

Chapter 7: Eat Like a Bodybuilder

1. Michael R. Lowe et al., "Dieting and Restrained Eating as Prospective Predictors of Weight Gain," *Frontiers in Psychology* 4 (2013): 577, https://www.ncbi.nlm.nih.gov/pmc/articles/PMC3759
019/.

2. Gary Taubes, "What Makes You Fat: Too Many Calories, or the Wrong Carbohydrates?," *Scientific American*, September 2013, https://www.scientificamerican.com/article/what-makes-you
-fat-too-many-calories-or-the-wrong-carbohydrates/.

3. Daniel E. Lieberman et al., "Comparing Measured Dietary Variation Within and Between Tropical Hunter-Gatherer Groups to the Paleo Diet," *American Journal of Clinical Nutrition* 118 (2023): 549–60, https://nme.fas.harvard.edu/sites/projects.iq.harvard.edu
/files/carmodylab/files/lieberman_et_al_2023_am_j_clin_nutr
.pdf.

4. "How Much Protein Do You Need Every Day?," Staying Healthy, Harvard Health Publishing, June 22, 2023, https://www.health

.harvard.edu/blog/how-much-protein-do-you-need-every-day -201506188096.

5. R. Jäger et al., "International Society of Sports Nutrition Position Stand: Protein and Exercise," *Journal of the International Society of Sports Nutrition* 14, no. 20 (2017), https://doi.org/10.1186/s12970-017-0177-8.

6. Barbara Davis, interview with the author, March 16, 2023.

7. Cell Press, "Eating Protein Boosts Hormone That Staves Off Hunger," ScienceDaily, September 6, 2006, https://www.sciencedaily.com/releases/2006/09/060905225848.htm.

8. H. J. Leidy et al., "The Influence of Higher Protein Intake and Greater Eating Frequency on Appetite Control in Overweight and Obese Men," *Obesity* (Silver Spring) 18, no. 9 (2010): 1725–32, http://doi.org/10.1038/oby.2010.45.

9. Kris Gunnars, "10 Science-Backed Reasons to Eat More Protein," Healthline, February 9, 2023, https://www.healthline.com/nutrition/10-reasons-to-eat-more-protein.

10. J. E. Kerstetter, A. M. Kenny, and K. L. Insogna, "Dietary Protein and Skeletal Health: A Review of Recent Human Research," *Curr Opin Lipidol* 22, no. 1 (2011): 16-20, https://doi.org/10.1097/MOL.0b013e3283419441.

11. J. I. Baum, I. Y. Kim, and R. R. Wolfe, "Protein Consumption and the Elderly: What Is the Optimal Level of Intake?," *Nutrients* 8, no. 6 (2016): 359, https://doi.org/10.3390/nu8060359.

12. Nina Teicholz, "A Short History of Saturated Fat: The Making and Unmaking of a Scientific Consensus," *Current Opinion in Endocrinology & Diabetes and Obesity* 30, no. 1 (2023): 65-71, https://doi.org/10.1097/MED.0000000000000079; "Higher Ratio of Plant Protein to Animal Protein May Improve Heart Health," Harvard T.H. Chan School of Public Health, December 2, 2024, https://hsph.harvard.edu/news/higher-ratio-of-plant-protein-to-animal-protein-may-improve-heart-health/.

13. Ashley N. Gearhardt et al., "Social, Clinical, and Policy Implications of Ultra-Processed Food Addiction," *BMJ* 383 (2023): e075354, https://www.bmj.com/content/383/bmj-2023-075354.

14. Kevin D. Hall et al., "Ultra-Processed Diets Cause Excess Calorie Intake and Weight Gain: An Inpatient Randomized Controlled Trial of *Ad Libitum* Food Intake," *Cell Metabolism* 30, no. 1 (2019): 67–77, E3, https://www.cell.com/cell-metabolism/fulltext/S1550 -4131(19)30248-7.

15. Paula Davis, "How the What-the-Hell Effect Impacts Your Will-power," *Psychology Today* (blog), January 31, 2017, https://www .psychologytoday.com/us/blog/pressure-proof/201701/how-the -what-the-hell-effect-impacts-your-willpower.

16. "Report Sets Dietary Intake Levels for Water, Salt, and Potassium to Maintain Health and Reduce Chronic Disease Risk," National Academies news release, https://www.nationalacademies.org /news/2004/02/report-sets-dietary-intake-levels-for-water-salt -and-potassium-to-maintain-health-and-reduce-chronic-disease -risk.

17. Mayo Clinic Staff, "Nutrition and Healthy Eating," Healthy Lifestyle, Mayo Clinic, October 12, 2022, https://www.mayoclinic .org/healthy-lifestyle/nutrition-and-healthy-eating/in-depth /water/art-20044256.

Epilogue

1. Paulina Porizkova (@paulinaporizkov), "To tan or not to tan . . . ," Instagram, March 15, 2024, https://www.instagram.com/p/C4jI CJtPsS-/.

2. Rachel Axon and Lindsay Schnell, "50 Years After Title IX Passed, Most Top Colleges Deprive Female Athletes of Equal Opportunities," *USA Today*, June 3, 2022, https://www.usatoday.com/in-depth/news /investigations/2022/06/03/title-ix-failures-50-years-colleges -women-lack-representation/9664260002/

INDEX